COVID Chronicles
How Essential
Workers Cope

———————

Therese Zink, MD, MPH

Published in the United States by **Zenterram Press**
ISBN: 978-0-9912651-6-9
Library of Congress Control Number: 2021906113
Cover Art and layout design: Reed Pike

All names and identifying characteristics have been altered to preserve anonymity or permission was granted. This is a work of creative nonfiction. In telling the stories of the individuals I interviewed, details may be altered and the timing of events collapsed so the book fits together as a whole and keeps the interest of readers.

DEDICATION

For all who suffered and continue to suffer in the COVID-19 pandemic. For those who cared for and continue to care for the suffering and try to make sense of it all.

Table of Contents

"It is now the very witching time . . . when churchyard yawn and hell itself breathing out Contagion to the world"
William Shakespeare, *Hamlet*, Act 3, Scene 2

Now gird up your loins . . .
Job 38:3

"The miserable have no other medicine, but only Hope."
William Shakespeare, *Measure for Measure*, Act 3, Scene 1

Introduction

The sun warmed my face that spring morning as I walked down the metal staircase, a short cut to avoid busy roads on my way to the University in Nablus, Palestine. Red, yellow, and lavender wild flowers sprang out amid the patches of green grass and piles of trash strewn across the hillside. After winter's rain, the desert was in bloom. As the recipient of a Fulbright award, I was a visiting faculty member in February and March 2020, teaching and mentoring at the medical school on the local university's campus.

A lanky Arab teenager who I'd passed other mornings stopped me half way. "Corona's here," he said in accented English.

"Corona?" He couldn't be referring to the Mexican beer. This was a conservative community in the heart of the West Bank, where alcohol was forbidden.

"Corona the virus."

"Shukran," I thanked him and continued on, smiling to myself. He was likely giving a general warning to the obvious foreigner who walked everywhere. This was not a walking culture, so I stood out without a hijab or dyed gray hair like most women my age.

I'd read about the virus cases in China, but this was the first report in the Middle East. When I reached the medical school, everyone knew that a South Korean church group visiting the holy sites had brought it to Bethlehem, and that they'd eaten knafah, a special sweet cheese dessert, in Nablus. It was only a matter of time.

Health officials quarantined the tourists in a Bethlehem hotel while one of the local doctors I worked with collected nasal swab tests from the visitors. She worried about her own exposure to the new virus, COVID-19. Within days, the group of local physicians I was teaching about Family Medicine began training on testing procedures and the proper use of masks and gowns, and some were called in to work extra shifts at the government clinics.

At the time, in the States, Seattle was reporting some cases, but my scan of the *New York Times* showed little about the new virus beyond the Wuhan epidemic and medical journals focused on the cases in China.

Within the week, Bethlehem locked down, and schools, mosques, and churches across the West Bank closed. Gatherings greater than 50 were prohibited. Foreigners became suspect, taxis refused to give rides, and a group of local teens spit at a black-skinned colleague. Our university host urged us to be careful.

There were no COVID cases in Nablus, so even though the university closed, I secured special permission from the dean to come into the medical school and wrap up projects with faculty. When we learned about a Palestinian physician who abandoned her patient in the exam room because the patient complained of a cough and fever, I helped local researchers launch a study on how doctors and nurses were coping with the new virus. This experience helped those professionals avoid fatigue as numbers grew; it would also prove invaluable to my later work during the pandemic.

A few kids who I'd passed many times during my walks through the neighborhood now yelled "foreigner" at me and giggled. I never felt afraid. However, as airlines out of Tel Aviv started canceling flights, the US embassy suggested we consider leaving. I did.

My flatmate and I packed quickly, arranging to leave several boxes in storage with colleagues at the university. The cleaning staff was delighted to have the labneh, tomatoes, and eggplant that remained in the refrigerator. With two months left in our commitment, we were sure we would return when this was over, with so much work remaining to be done in our Fulbright commitments. When the COVID mess was all over, I thought, I'd find myself some Corona beer and Mexican food and figure out how to celebrate. Little did I know.

A few people on the packed plane wore masks and disinfected their seats with alcohol wipes, but I was not one of them. In fact, during the 12-hour flight, I looked askance at those nervous ninnies. At this point, only people from Asia wore masks, probably because of the horrible air pollution in their large cities. There was no scientific evidence that I knew of that reported masks to do anything but make one feel claustrophobic—little did I know how rapidly my perspective would change.

Arriving at JFK, my connecting flight was too tight to make. I just wanted to get home, so I skipped the flight and caught the train to Rhode Island. COVID hadn't yet shut down New York City, but Penn Station was creepily empty, another warning of what was to come. The Amtrak ride up the coast made for a pleasant reentry. I dozed and watched the sun drenched coastal towns and harbors on the mid-March afternoon, mulling over recent experiences in Palestine: The new virus. The fear and uncertainty of the physicians and nurses. The worries about adequate gowns and masks. The targeting of dark-skinned people and foreigners. The additional challenges of managing as an occupied state where the occupier, Israel, set the rules. Checkpoints were under the control of Israel and closures had affected the route I took to the airport.

Finally, I arrived home after nearly 24 hours en route. I was a month earlier than expected after only six weeks abroad, and little did I know that I was walking into a Michael Crichton pandemic thriller.

The day after I passed through JFK airport, the passport control lines were hours long due to newly implemented health screenings. Some passengers spent over eight hours in line further increasing their exposure to COVID. Although I didn't think I had contracted the virus, I followed advice given by the CDC to foreign travelers and self-quarantined for two weeks.

Soon I was listening to the weekly Rhode Island Department of Health phone calls for physicians and watching National Academy of Medicine podcasts to learn the science about the novel SARS-CoV-2 or COVID-19 virus. My medical career was overshadowed by AIDS in the 1980s and now COVID-19 in 2020. As interns in the 80s, we were always trying to understand the new disease—AIDS. We instituted universal precautions, using gloves when in contact with body fluids, taking special precautions after needle pricks. At the time, death from HIV was a forgone conclusion for those infected, but over the decades, researchers learned more about the virus and the human immune system. Better tests for monitoring the body's response and new drugs were developed. HIV has come to be treated as a chronic disease. With COVID the possibility of illness or death began to surface everywhere as part of the job and a constant underlying concern.

Within days, the US and the world changed around me.

Soon, I wouldn't think of leaving home without a mask: research showed it was imperative to prevent the spread of the virus, whose primary vector, or communicability, was airborne particles. And I wouldn't leave home unless I had to. Doctors and healthcare facilities struggled to procure protective equipment. I would begin to understand how the color of one's skin predicted a greater chance of catching the virus and the severity of the illness.

Of course, we already know something about this story. The US and the world are still wading through a once in a century pandemic. Millions die, others recover, and some, known as long haulers, are plagued with continuing problems. Due to the contagion, people are unable to comfort each other. Some choose not to heed advice and spread the virus, feeling it is more important to exercise their rights of personal freedom. National leaders falter and some scoff at science.

Caring for the sick has taxed my profession and my coping skills as I watch coworkers, patients, and families stretched thin and taut like rubber bands ready to snap. And beyond healthcare, there are other essential workers, people who do the grunt work of the world—cooks, cleaners, drivers, food preparers, police.

These Chronicles of mine explore how essential workers fared and coped during the first year. How they negotiated a way forward in the chaos of the crisis, moved from darkness into light. We will explore some of the critical lessons, and the discussions we must have as a society if we don't want to relive these struggles when the next novel virus appears in our global world. Finally, let's acknowledge the essential workers who accepted the risk and sacrificed their lives to keep the world moving forward.

Although I am gray haired and the struggles with COVID-19 will stretch beyond my years of doctoring, I am heartened by the courage and new energy and perspectives of the next generation of caregivers and essential workers. The perspectives I encountered in my workday encouraged me to go searching for other stories. I found them across the country—from other doctors, medical assistants, customer service workers, and school nurses. Closer to home, I watched my own family struggle and survive. I rode a roller coaster of emotions and wrote my way into understanding how to cope and make sense of all that swirled around me.

Most interviews were done virtually thanks to today's technologies. Some interviewees allowed me to use their first names; others preferred a pseudonym. Exact locations are not shared to protect the privacy of those I spoke with as well as the patients, relatives, or clients discussed. Writing in the genre of creative nonfiction, I have not recounted every detail. At times events are compressed, but I have tried to render the essence of the experiences, feelings and musings of those I interviewed and to portray the vitality and resilience they bring to these difficult times. Let's celebrate the hope this next generation brings to life's inevitable cycle. May you also find your own way forward and your own beacons of promise.

Chapter 1 — Therese

My Story: Too Many Birthday Candles

"You have too many birthday candles to treat COVID patients."

My shoulders tightened and the phone slipped in my sweaty palm as I absorbed my boss's words.

I started to argue. I had taken an oath. I owed it to my colleagues to stand in the trenches, to do my part, to share the burden of risk.

But I would be 65 in Fall 2020. I had high blood pressure. I didn't want to get sick, nor die. I didn't want to expose my family. And most of all I didn't want to spend weeks in the ICU and cause anguish to my loved ones, or suffer the many potential complications.

"We need your expertise with telehealth," he said.

Something like relief caught in my chest. "Okay," I said. He was stroking my ego, but frankly, he was right and he'd given me an out. But guilt returned every time I watched television replays of New Yorkers saluting their health care heroes nightly at 7 p.m., leaning out of brick buildings clapping, waving signs, banging metal pans, as church bells chimed the hour.

Due to the pandemic, insurance companies finally agreed to pay for virtual visits now that the medical profession had struggled to implement that mode of patient care for the last ten years. But payment and legal issues were hard to iron out with health insurers. COVID changed everything. The worry of infectious spread was a no-brainer. It's more convenient for patients—no time-off work, making plans for the kids, climbing in a car, or waiting for the bus. Good internet access was a problem for our low-income patients, so telehealth was via phone, without fancy video equipment. If I needed to see a rash, I asked the patient to text me a photo.

That first Saturday morning in spring, I sat at my dining room table and opened my laptop. Forty-some COVID test results sat in my inbox and more than three-quarters were positive. My job was to call each patient, give the result, and explain the current CDC (Center for Disease Control & Prevention) guidance on how to stay safe, how to manage the symptoms, the rules of quarantine, and when to call us or 911.

I swallowed a swig of coffee. As an oldest child and a physician for 30 plus years, I was good at telling people what to do.

"Hello Ms. S, this is Dr. Zink at Providence Clinic. I have your COVID test result. You speak English?"

"*Si, si,*" she said in accented English.

"You are positive for COVID."

"Oh dear."

"Who lives with you?"

"My husband, four children and my mother-in-law."

"Is anyone else sick?"

"No. Should they be tested?"

"Not until they develop symptoms. You need to try to isolate yourself from them. Can you stay in a room by yourself?"

"That's hard. We only have three rooms and one bathroom."

"You should wear a mask when you are around them, and clean the bathroom before and after you use it. Someone else should do the cooking. Is that possible?"

"That'll be difficult."

"I realize that." I bit at my lip.

"I can't sleep with my husband?"

"No. I'm sorry."

"That means I'm sleeping on the couch."

"Maybe you stay in the bedroom and he takes the couch."

"He won't do that," she sighed.

I quickly appreciated the sheer challenge of what we were asking people to do.

Early on, there weren't enough tests so we prioritized them. "We can't test you unless you have symptoms which include: fever, sore throat, cough," I told a city bus driver.

"I feel fine. So no tests until I feel sick?"

"That's what we're doing now, but that might change. Call us if you have questions."

And it did change. It was hard to keep up. I printed out protocols for quick reference, and stored others on my laptop. I updated them frequently. It was confusing for patients and hence, hard to inspire confidence and trust.

"Señora, you do not have COVID. Your test was negative."

"Oh, really, I feel lousy."

"Well other things can make you feel sick."

"But I've lost my sense of taste and smell."

"Patients frequently complain of that, but those symptoms aren't on the list." (They were added later on.)

"But my husband is COVID positive, so I can't believe I'm not."

"Well, the test isn't perfect. Sometimes we get false negatives. We're still learning and developing better tests." I squirmed in my chair, and apologized for the confusion.

"What should I do?"

After reviewing mask wearing, handwashing and social distancing, I asked, "Does your phone receive text messages? I'll send you a link to a health department information page which summarizes what I just told you…"

I felt helpless, trying to make the complex instructions easier. Maybe if they read it! I survived on the occasional thank you or gracias.

Fantasy treatments and outright lies filled the news.

"No, don't drink bleach or Lysol," I warned a forty-something male. I wanted to stick pins into a voodoo doll with orange hair.

"No, there is no treatment. Your cousin in Mexico may have been given an antibiotic, but we aren't allowed to do that here. You can't treat a virus with antibiotics. Your body makes proteins…"

He wanted a magic bullet. He wasn't happy with me.

The hardest conversations were with those who had lost a job and were the household's only source of income. Or they were COVID positive and shouldn't work, but had to. I shared food bank resources and connected them with the social worker, so grateful that the clinic offered some help negotiating unemployment, gas, and electric payment support, especially for non-English speakers. My heart twisted and my mouth grew dry; it wasn't enough.

Silently, I counted my own blessings and berated myself for my own pity parties.

"I am so nervous, I can't sleep," a patient said in a tight voice.

I assessed for depression and arranged for behavioral health to call.

"I am short of breath sometimes…"

He didn't gasp as he spoke, so I didn't call 911. Instead, I arranged an appointment in the respiratory assessment clinic an hour later. There, staff in masks, face shields, gloves, and gowns would assess his temperature and oxygen levels, and listen to his lungs. If the oxygen level was low, the patient was directed to Emergency. If all was fine, staff sent the results to me.

By the end of my four hours, I slouched, exhausted and overwhelmed by how hard this virus was for people, especially people who lived paycheck to paycheck, or rather two paychecks to two paychecks, essential workers who didn't have sick time.

As I shut down my laptop, I was ashamed of my own irritation at being stuck at home. No movies, closed restaurants, no concerts or theater, no travel, no visits to the gym to swim or workout for me.

Every telehealth shift reminded me that I had nothing to complain about. It was also clear that the stats were right — brown- and black-skinned people, who were a high percentage of my patients, were disproportionately affected and the impact went beyond just being ill. But it was hard to know precisely where to direct my anger. There were a lot of possibilities. And little did I know how horrible it would become, especially when my sister and mother contracted COVID.

Chapter 2 — Ben

Inside the Testing Tent

As a podiatrist, Dr. Ben usually focuses on feet. But years of military service and his expertise in program implementation and measurement qualified him to set up a COVID test site in Spring 2020. Testing stations were available in the suburbs, but the heart of the pandemic, the urban center, needed a walk-up and drive-up option. The medical director of the network of low-income clinics tasked him with the job. Together they watched the National Guard's testing video and read the pertinent CDC guidelines.

"We can't spare a nurse to assist you," the medical director said.

"I'll figure it out. Give me the weekend. Start scheduling appointments for Monday."

Dr. Ben disappeared into his basement workshop to create a contraption to support a "solo COVID tester."

Two wooden testing platforms, each a little bigger than a cutting board, one painted white and the other blue, secured parts of the specimen kit—tube, cap, plastic bag with requisition and swab—so they wouldn't roll or blow away. The platforms sat on a rectangular table inside the tent along with boxes of gloves, a bottle of hand sanitizer, and a Styrofoam container holding a bag of ice. Cars and people queued in the alley, checked in with the receptionist at a kiosk who tucked the kit and requisition under the windshield wiper or hand carried it to the tent. Either patients' noses were swabbed in their cars with the window rolled halfway down, or they took a seat in a plastic chair inside the tent.

"Please put your car in park," I said. *"Parque."* I didn't want to risk a foot slipping off the brake when sticking a long Q-tip into someone's nose. I incorporated Dr. Ben's first lesson for me. By the time I joined him in December, he'd collected over a thousand tests. In his outdoor tent, he'd managed the chill of Spring 2020, and the scorching Summer. Now as winter approached, he was retiring from this task and training a squad of testing newbies. I was one of them.

The first challenge was putting on Personal Protective Equipment (PPE). When swabbing patient after patient who have COVID symptoms, it was important not to infect yourself or someone else.

Donning PPE is a novelty the first time and YouTube videos demonstrate the many steps. If you've done it, you likely have your own funny anecdotes. The first task is to secure the materials (gown, gloves, and mask) in the correct sizes. If your shoes can't be cleaned with alcohol wipes, then you need shoe covers too. After pulling the one-size fits-all paper version over your shoes, be sure to wash your hands with sanitizer.

Next, the paper gown is worn over clothes, often hospital-style scrubs. If it's cold weather, long underwear is essential. If it's summer, remember even a paper gown holds in some heat; so dress accordingly. The hair cover does what the name suggests, and the face shield or googles protect the eyes because the virus can enter through the mucous membranes around the eyes. The protection is a reminder not to touch your face, something we all do. Pulling on gloves follows and the first pair goes over your gown's cuffs. Depending on what you are doing, you may wear additional layers of gloves. It's a struggle to pull on the final pairs each time after having doused the second pair in sanitizer. As a whole, gloving is the most time consuming and frustrating part of the process, and nerve wracking as patients wait patiently or not so patiently for you to complete the antic.

As a clinician working with patients who may be infected with COVID, I was pre-fitted for the N95 respirator mask. It requires a special session to ensure a tight seal so that airborne particles cannot enter. The fitter sprays sweetened air into a plastic head cover that sits like an astronaut's helmet on the fitee's shoulders. You breathe, talk, read a poem, and bend over to make sure you can't taste sweetness during any of the maneuvers. WARNING: If the mask is too tight, which was my problem for the first week, you will find yourself talking like a ventriloquist.

The Bureau of Mines and the National Institute for Occupational Safety and Health (NIOSH) teamed up to create the first "dust" respirators before the 1970s. 3M developed the single-use N95, first approved in 1972. But in 1992, researchers at the University of Tennessee added an electrostatic charge inside the mask that makes it breathable, but keeps viral particles out, and voilá the modern N95 respirator mask used widely today in health care facilities around the world.

Note: The KN95 has the electrostatic charge, but does not meet NIOSH standards. Many are manufactured in China and can be purchased off the internet and in stores like Walmart and Home Depot. It provides more respiratory protection than a cloth face mask or surgical mask when working in clinical settings. Currently, the CDC recommends that the public wear a simple two-layer cloth face mask that covers the nose and mouth. Neck gaiters are folded in two layers and bandanas don't count. But watch the CDC web site, it could change.

Many have experienced the COVID test. Some might accuse testers of trying to tickle the brain, or shoving a roto-rooter up a nostril. The process is definitely fodder for the late night comedians.

Collecting the test takes some skill, and eye-hand coordination. As gently as possible, I reach a flexible Q-tip into a nostril and push it to where the nose meets the throat—the oropharynx. Eyes water, some people gag, others sneeze. Ideally, the patient holds still and doesn't jerk their head, grab your hand, or squirm their body away. However, all reactions are to be expected.

Dr. Ben kept a record of his observations. He calls the COVID nasal test the great equalizer. He knew the swabbing didn't hurt but was discomforting to everyone: Eyes water at the very least. Girls aged eight to ten are the bravest, sitting still and afterwards quietly wiping away the tears running down the face.

Tough, city gang kids try to be cool but grunt out the hurt, "Wow, man, where did you go with that?"

One twenty-something had a roll of money in his lap, smelled of pot, but was the model of politeness: "Thank you, doctor."

After Ben collected a specimen from a fellow with tattoos and chains, the tough fellow warned, "I'm jumping out of my car to punch you in the face for that." Instead, Tattoos gunned his Prius and sped away.

A couple rolled up in an old Honda. The husband, who was driving, went first and yelled, "Take it out, take it out!" as he white-knuckled the steering wheel. The wife smiled after watching her husband and said, "I really enjoyed that," before submitting to her own swabbing.

My most delightful patient was a four-year-old who sat on her mother's lap. I entice all children telling them this will tickle. "*Giggle, giggle.*" This little girl heard my suggestion and her chirp lightened the procedure for her mother and me.

To distract kids, I give them a pair of latex gloves as a souvenir, or ask the parent to blow a glove into a balloon. *Voila!* A funny looking monster's head to play with.

On Ben's final day, a six-year-old boy, who sat in the chair, shot out his leg as the swab went into his nose. Ben jumped back with a yelp. You can guess where the boy's foot made contact: yup, his groin. Good-natured Ben considered it his farewell send off, and had a good laugh. I am guessing he's retold that story a few times.

We passed the time listening to Ben's Spotify, a sampling of 70s, 80s, and 90s hits. He played to the requests of his squad in training. We made jokes about mask-wearing styles: chin straps, mustaches, earrings, bracelets, and headbands. The newest rear-view mirror ornaments. And we groaned about masks as the new litter. We complained about our fogged up glasses and hoarse voices from yelling in order to be heard.

His great sense of humor reminded me that finding the funny in all of this was a way to cope. While joking during this once-in-a-century pandemic may seem inappropriate to some, it is an essential ingredient for survival.

Finally, when the mask is growing uncomfortably tight, after the last appointment, we count specimen bags and make sure our numbers jive with the registrar's list. If not, get ready for comparing requisitions, specimen tubes, and the appointment list. No fun!

Removing PPE, or doffing, is a bit more challenging than putting it on and is usually done while standing inside a trash bag. You step into the large red bag—don't put it over your head. Shoe covers, or what remains intact after treading around on asphalt for four hours, are torn apart, and you step out of them. An outer glove is peeled off, exposing the glove inside. Tuck one inside the other. The gown is ripped and pulled forward, and rolled down then thrown into the trash bag—sort of reminiscent of a bodice-ripping thriller except you are doing it to yourself.

Remove another glove layer, then the hairnet, face shield, or goggles, and outer face mask; discard all into the bag. Step out of it, rolling and tying it shut. The N95 is taken off without touching the mask's front, which may be coated with virus particles. Store it in a paper bag until the next use. Keeping it in your pocket is a no-no. Hands are washed. One jokester chided, "I never imagined my hands would consume more alcohol than my mouth."

Now try to do the entire process quickly and imaging dressing up and down, multiple times a day. It takes about five minutes to put it on and at least another five to take it off. Note: procedures may vary at different health care facilities. And there were moments when I wondered if four gloves were too much given that some countries wash and reuse their gloves to have enough. But alas.

Ingenious Dr. Ben decided it was time to "retire" from testing as winter rumbled in. Enough of the cold toes despite the heater blowing at your feet and up the gown. His wife, with an autoimmune condition, was also encouraging him to return to his usual day job. Ben had more than done his duty and created and shepherded a smooth operation into the third surge. It was time to take care of himself and his family.

Ben's contribution reminds me that dealing with the crisis of the pandemic requires being creative, matching skills to tasks, and often reassigning staff. Ben revived the old adage of "thinking outside the box to solve the problems" for this pandemic. Stepping up and into new roles is never easy, but a good manager sees what needs to be done, finds the right people to lead and perform the duties, and then encourages with vision and humor.

I've taken over Dr. Ben's Friday mornings, having had my first vaccination, or "jab" as they call it in Britain. Dressed up in layers of PPE, and with more knowledge about COVID, I feel safer now facing the virus months later. I value the ability to do my part in these difficult times. When the swabbing becomes a grind, and patients' responses are annoying, I think of Dr. Ben and his jokes. And I wish I were funnier.

Chapter 3 — Anna

A Full-Bore Sprint

The ICU throbbed day and night at full speed in the East coast city. There was no warmup or cool-down, just a full-bore sprint. Patients were sick, very sick. Ventilators hissed, HEPA air purifiers whirred, and machines clicked as they pumped fluids and medicines through tubes into patients. Even though she was early in her career as an internal medicine physician, finishing her residency training, Dr. Anna did not cower. Despite appearing small boned and fragile, she was up to the task.

The ICU was not new to her. She'd spent time there pre-COVID when patients were sick, but not so sick that everyone needed a ventilator. Then families could stay with their loved ones day and night, and she was grateful for those days: "We got to know the patients and their families. When we had difficult conversations, such as end of life discussions—'your mom has taken a turn for the worse'—families trusted us. You could be gentle, and if they missed the subtlety, you could be more direct later in the day. They knew we were working hard because they sat in the room and watched us. They could see the decline in their loved ones and watch the monitors. We could revisit the tough conversations, help family members work through the horrible realities of loss, medical interventions that weren't working."

With COVID, the ICU was packed and every patient lay prone, flat with their chest down on the bed, as ventilators helped them breathe. The most astonishing fact to Dr. Anna was that patients were much younger, in their 40s and 50s, the same ages as some of the nurses and physicians in charge. Patients who should have been in ICU were moved on to other floors because the ICU didn't have space. Dr. Anna and her team knew their patients because they had cared for them for weeks. Family photos and artwork by grandkids and kids decorated the walls. But no family members were physically present. It was too dangerous with COVID, but absence presented other difficulties: "We zoomed routinely with family. But it's hard to read body language on Zoom, and they weren't watching us work hour after hour caring for their mother, daughter, son, or husband. They couldn't see how awful their loved ones looked. When things took a turn, we had to be direct. Sometimes it felt harsh. That was hard to get used to."

One of the worst cases she tended was the father of a young family. Chad was admitted with COVID and needed a ventilator. He seemed to be showing some improvement and Anna and her team were hopeful. Then suddenly he took a turn for the worse, his need for oxygen increased, suggesting that he had blood clots in his lungs, a common scenario with severe COVID cases. On Father's Day, he coded—he had a heart attack and his heart stopped. Anna said, "I had to call his wife, on Father's Day of all days. I could hear their kids playing in the background. She was shocked and kept asking why we didn't know this was going to happen. It was terrible, she kept second-guessing us—what did we miss, what did we do wrong? If she'd been in the room, she would have seen that her husband was getting sicker and sicker despite everything we were doing. There were lots of unhappy endings in the ICU, patients died, despite all our efforts."

Anna told me that the nurses had it the hardest because they knew the patients and their families the best. They cared for one or two patients at a time, and were assigned to the same patient whenever they worked in the ICU. That meant weeks with the same patient, hour after hour at the bedside, while the doctors hurried from patient to patient to oversee their care, review test results and labs, and write orders for dozens and dozens of very sick people.

A study showed that the safest way to deploy physicians during training who were working with COVID patients was in a seven-days on and seven-days off cycle. That gave enough time for physicians to show the signs or symptoms of COVID or have a test turn positive so they wouldn't return to work and infect their colleagues. To make this work, the hospital rearranged schedules and pulled in residents in other specialties who volunteered to help. This meant that dermatology, pathology, and radiology residents and fellows joined ICU teams as junior doctors to help oversee patient care. Some were suddenly back on wards after a year or more in the lab or clinic—not an easy task, but everyone pitched in. One of the attendings, the physician in charge of the team who was also retired military, emphasized "survival by pulling together in the trenches." Anna said, "His approach created tremendous camaraderie despite the challenge and we found reasons to laugh together."

Humor and funny stories helped everyone cope: "You can't be sad and overwhelmed day in and day out." Anna describes laughing about a pet or partner's antics. One colleague lightened the mood with pranks. One evening Anna's beeper paged her to call Dr. Berger about a patient named Wendy. When Anna dialed the number, and said, "I'm answering a page from Dr. Berger," the person on the other end replied, "This is Wendy's Restaurant. We don't have a Dr. Berger here."

Anna clicked off her phone and chuckled—Dr. Prankster hit again.

When the new residents joined the daily rounds at the beginning of their ICU rotation, one took Anna aside and whispered, "The team seemed really flippant about the patients this morning. How can you crack jokes with so many ill patients, some dying. It seems disrespectful."

"I'm sorry," Anna said. "Rounds are heavy, 18 intubated and prone patients, everyone very sick. If we waited for lighter times, we would never joke at all. We can't be sad and depressed all the time."

The intern listened and then grew quiet. A few days later, she brought in a comic strip depicting the same situation. "She got it," Anna told me, adding, "Humor allows you to gown and suit up and show up each day to face the tragedy of patients who are struggling for their lives. It helps face the desperation of families, witnessed on Zoom. Families, who wanted to be present to comfort their loved ones, and could not. And face the reality that you run the risk of catching the virus despite all your caution, especially when the nation's leadership isn't taking it seriously. Humor helps you face the fact that some people were dissing the profession to which you had committed your life."

In the beginning, PPE was a problem. Since there was no national coordinated effort, the states were on their own. Anna's hospital donated 300,000 N95 masks to a neighboring state that was in crisis. When the COVID numbers began to climb at home, PPE was scarce. The state was promised a truckload of PPE, but it arrived empty. A local engineering school began producing N95 masks on 3D printers. Local efforts to procure PPE were eventually successful, but Anna says it was hard to be on the living end of the scarcity while numbers were climbing.

She was given one N95 mask to wear for her five weeks in the ICU. While she wore a paper mask over it to protect it, she sweated and sneezed, intubated patients, and was sprayed with body fluids: "I remember adjusting the mask as I walked to the bedside of a very sick patient and thinking, Here we go. I hope this dirty thing is still protecting me. It was nerve wracking, you just didn   t know. One day I got blood on it and needed a new one."

That time, Anna had to stay after her night shift to go to the mask allocation site. The limited hours were appointment only, so she signed her name and the reason she needed a new mask: "It felt like I'd done something wrong. Like I could have prevented getting sprayed with blood." Thankfully, she only had to go through that once.

PPE became more plentiful when the hospital purchased plastic masks with changeable filters. They muffled voices even more, but could be cleaned. Anna loved to talk, but her higher frequency voice was hard to hear under all the PPE: "If the nurses couldn't hear me when I yelled, I wrote things down. That doesn't work very well in an emergency."

This may be the new normal for Anna and this generation of health care workers, especially with the growing number of COVID-19 mutations that are highly contagious and may not respond to the vaccines.

Anna felt proud to be part of a residency program that modeled great leadership and to have a supportive partner at home: "I compared notes with classmates in other parts of the country. Hands down, I am glad I'm working where I am during the pandemic." The program excelled at infection management, and they changed the schedule to minimize the chance of asymptomatic exposure. Communication included a daily email updating the residents on the PPE situation, the number of patients in the hospital, the number of patients on ventilators, and resident schedules. Rotations changed constantly. Elective rotations were canceled and more residents were allocated to cover the hospital wards. Clinics moved to telehealth. "Things were constantly changing," she said, "but they kept us up on the latest. It was a great comfort."

A psychologist held a weekly zoom session for the residents to provide a safe space to commiserate. "We knew we weren't alone with what we were feeling," Anna acknowledged. The psychologist offered individual sessions as well: "One of the most helpful discussions was about boundary setting," as many residents were the go-to-source of medical information for their families and friends: "It was a daunting responsibility and the therapist helped us say, 'I can't talk today, but maybe later.' We all needed permission to say, 'No, not right now, I'm sorry. It's been a bad day.'"

The other great advice was to come home and do something else before going to sleep, despite the exhaustion. "She encouraged us to give our brains a break for even a little bit," Anna said. "My cat got a lot of playtime." Anna also read fiction to decompress.

"Usually I am someone who talks to process my day, share the stories. But that didn't work with COVID. I couldn't relive all the difficult experiences. My partner got that. He would let me be. But he listened when I was ready to talk. We cooked together, simple recipes. We watched movies and television together. Everybody talked about *Tiger King*. Then there was *Schitt's Creek*, *The Good Place*, and *Mindhunter*." Anna treasures having a partner and can't imagine having to come home to an empty apartment: "Being solely responsible for laundry, cleaning, and the dishes would have been hard."

When Dr. Anna and her partner masked up to make a grocery store run during the peak of the first COVID surge, they saw unmasked individuals barging into the store. Her fury burned. "How deeply arrogant to believe that you don't need to protect yourself and others," she said. "Wearing a mask is the smallest ask."

Chapter 4 — Jasmine

The Dysfunction Magnified

Jasmine wears many hats: caregiver at a group home in a rural county, full-time student at a community college, housemate for her mother, and sister to two teenage brothers who are struggling with distance learning. "This is a challenging time" is an understatement, coming from her, although a frown rarely ripples across Jasmine's face. Her how are you feels sincere, not the routine greeting that expects a just fine response. She is honestly interested in how your day has been, and whether or not an ill loved one is doing better. And she cares deeply about her clients. Her lap creates a comfortable nest for the small nonverbal twenty-something at the group home who constantly asks for soda pop; Jasmine calmly redirects her in a soft alto tone and offers reassurance. They're about the same age.

Then there is Stacy who is twice their age and loves to stay up late. She sits in her wheelchair at her desk calling family and friends as she watches television. "Stacy, it's 10 p.m., it's past your bedtime. What will your sister say?" Jasmine asks, rubbing Stacy's shoulders.

"I don't believe that," Stacy says and looks at her clock. "It's 9:57."

Jasmine stifles a chuckle and gives Stacy her medications, then deftly coaxes her toward bed. Staying up is one of the few actions Stacy can control.

Although Jasmine works in health care, she hopes to study

law. She works full-time to pay tuition and the bills at home, the
home she shares with her mother and brothers. However, her
experience with special needs adults will serve her well in the
legal profession, especially if she represents clients with disabili-
ties or mental health challenges. "Every experience is useful and
difficult ones just make you stronger and smarter," she claims,
her voice carrying the tenor of a sage.

"COVID makes everything harder," Jasmine told me. "It magnifies the dysfunction." Virtual classes in criminal justice were
okay, some teachers managed better than others, and the college offered students decent support with the online platform.
Things fell apart when she tried to secure work experience in
the legal setting: "That's hard to set up virtually. There are many
more hoops to jump through, more gates to open and close in
order to secure an interview." Mentors were reluctant to oversee a student and expose themselves and their office to infection. Jasmine had to figure out where to get a COVID test, and
assuming she tested negative, she emailed the result and tried to
schedule an appointment for a day that the law office was open,
squeezing in between her full-time school and work schedules.
"At the interview, I have to be my very best. I worry, practice,
and rehearse possible questions." Even today, for a black girl,
attending a community college with the goal of law school was
a stretch, and COVID turned it into a pole vault.

"Disappointed" was how Jasmine felt about the response of the
powers that be to the pandemic: disappointed in her supervisors
at the group home facilities, disappointed with administration
at the nursing home where her mother works, disappointed in
the state health department, disappointed in the educators at
the public high school her brothers attend, and disappointed in
national leadership.

Jasmine puts her all into everything she does. She's the person you would want on your team, the caregiver you want caring for your child or parent. She feels responsible for the welfare of the women in the group home and gives 150 percent.

Her supervisor expects her to come in and work on her day off, when help is needed. Even before COVID there were slackers, and supervisors failed to address the underperformers. With COVID the problems and poor management were magnified. Jasmine told me she worries clients are at risk because frontline workers aren't careful about what they do on their own time. Masks were not required at work and protocols about working when sick were not taken seriously. "Administration should do better." She folded her arms across her chest and her forehead wrinkled. "The county and state should hold them to higher standards. We are caring for vulnerable adults."

When Jasmine's mother turned up COVID positive on a routine screen at the nursing home where she works as a nurse's assistant, Jasmine dutifully called her supervisor at the group home. "I think I need to quarantine and get a test," she said. "I live with my Mom who has COVID."

"No worries, we need you here," the supervisor said. "If you aren't feeling sick, come on in. We check temperatures."

For a moment, Jasmine fell silent. Some of the clients had medical problems like asthma and obesity. If she made them sick, she'd never forgive herself. "Well, okay," she said. "Are you sure?"

"We need you here."

Jasmine took it upon herself to secure a test, even though the supervisor didn't ask for one. She owed it to herself, her brothers, as well as her coworkers and the clients at the group home. And she wore a mask, even though it wasn't required. The COVID rates weren't as high in the rural county where she worked as they were in the nearby urban area, so group home administrators decided not to enforce the state's mask-wearing mandates in the rural homes.

"When I tested negative, I whispered a thank you prayer to God," she said and blessed herself. Should Jasmine have contracted COVID, she had additional risks due to obesity and her race/ethnicity. The obese are at risk for a more severe illness. Blacks have a greater chance of dying from COVID (Black versus White, 2:1) and three times the rate of hospitalization.

Jasmine's mother reported many of the same concerns at work: supplies like gloves, masks and gowns are inadequate and nursing home administrators haven't secured them. "It infuriates both of us," Jasmine said and added, "Administrators are not on the front lines and they don't understand what their employees are facing. We are putting ourselves at risk."

Jasmine and her mother expected more than a vicious cycle of staff infecting patients and visa versa. In addition, both complained that the state had not stepped in: "They do their checks; write their reports. At the time they come through the facility, all looks fine, and they don't dig any deeper. Rarely do officials interview frontline staff to see what's going on, and if they do, staff worry about losing their jobs if they are honest."

Jasmine is right. National Public Radio and other news organizations have reported the woefully inadequate supplies in some nursing homes. Most nursing homes are chronically understaffed and it has only grown worse with the pandemic. Staff often work sick because the pay is low, health insurance is not covered, or partially covered, and sick time is not paid or only available after a certain number work hours. Many nursing assistants work two jobs, sometimes in two different facilities to make ends meet. COVID has marched through nursing homes, and staff and residents in long-term care facilities represented 40 percent of the US deaths due to COVID at the end of 2020. Over 400,000 died of COVID during 2020; more than 160,000 in long-term care facilities.

While facility administrators and state officials may be at fault, blame also goes to the lack of national leadership. Because PPE planning, purchasing, and distribution were not organized at the national level, the authority under the Defense Production Act to secure adequate supplies was never enacted, states and individual facilities ended up scrambling on their own during 2020. Without clear guidelines and mandates at the national level, PPE procurement was delegated to a variety of actors: state and city governments, large hospital chains, and in some cases small networks of clinics. Some did well, others failed miserably and city and county officials were forced to step in in but had little power to effectively find resources or wield much authority. In addition, the US government disassembled previous efforts to prepare for pandemics after Hurricane Katrina, H1N1 and Ebola due to ignorance, budget issues, politics, and other priorities.

Jasmine's disappointment in her employers and her government also underlined the chronic neglect and inattention to the welfare of people with black and brown skin. While people who look like her were faring poorly in the pandemic, much worse than whites, it's been the norm for centuries. In fact, the protests that surfaced after the death of George Floyd which coincided with the pandemic highlighted the centuries of inequities in the US due to race and skin color.

Jasmine also worried that her teenage brothers in public high school were victims of the same injustice. Both had a difficult time with home schooling. One was into sports but all team activities were on hold. Hence he missed his social circle and physical activity, an important outlet for him. Her other brother was unmotivated to do his computer schoolwork.

"When I'm home, I remind him to get on line and do his studies. We have good internet, so that isn't the problem. He looks at me and goes back to his video games. He's bigger than me. I can't make him. My mom can't either. Video games, that's all he does, night and day," she worried.

Jasmine blamed the school's administration for failing to address the psychological preparation needed to do online work and for never teaching self-management skills. "They quickly transitioned and pushed out the academics. They offered nothing to help the students manage this new way of learning, no follow-up to see how they're coping," she sighed, and then told me, "I worry about their future and their peers. Can they recover a lost year when finishing up high school? Can they get decent jobs? They are black men. They already have many counts against them." Jasmine wondered if it might be different at a private school. Was her brother's school written off because it was public with a largely black student body?

These are big questions. Heavy burdens to bear when you are in your early twenties.

I asked Jasmine how she copes.

"Faith and scripture keep me going," she said and shared a passage from Proverbs: *Trust in the Lord with all your heart; do not depend on your own understanding. Seek His will in all you do and He will show you which path to take* (Proverbs 3:5-6).

"God has His ways. I just need to believe." Jasmine continued, "It can be very depressing, but I am able to have a difficult moment and realize that I can rise above it. I cannot change it. It is what it is and complaining and being depressed just makes it harder. I try to be positive. It is easier to be positive. Faith and being a child of God makes it easier. I start by really caring for and about people."

I asked Jasmine her thoughts about the vaccine.

She said she prefers to wait a little while and not be in the first group. The artificial components of the vaccine concerned her, as well as reports of allergic reactions. We discussed the history of distrusting medicine among Blacks—with the terrible legacy of Tuskegee and radiation exposure experiments. She worried how the vaccine will be rolled out in prisons where inmates are largely black. Her criminal justice background came through as she pointed out that private prisons have less oversight than state or federal facilities, and what that means for inmate rights. She hoped that someone who looks like her was part of the scientific team that developed the vaccine. (In fact, Dr. Anthony Fauci and others have highlighted the female African American scientist, Dr. Kizzmekia Corbett, who was on the NIH team.)

Our society has a long way to go to address the history of inequality and structural discrimination of black and brown people that were and continue to be the foundation of our country. For the first time in recent history, nonviolent demonstrations have been composed of large numbers of white-skinned people alongside the black and brown-skinned protestors. Perhaps we are moving toward more justice and fairness for all.

Jasmine is one of those individuals who is determined to overcome that previous history.

Her mother's and her descriptions of the shortcomings of the administration and government during this pandemic should concern all of us. The impact those shortcomings have had on the elderly and special needs patients in care facilities, prisoners, students, the unemployed and underemployed during this pandemic are tragic and perhaps even criminal. In fact, the impacts are underestimated and will have significant long-term impacts on our future. Hopefully, Jasmine will have and be given the opportunity to be part of the solution—we can only hope!

Chapter 5 — Alan

Fighting Two Wars

A trainee just back from an international vacation gave Dr. Alan COVID-19. "I thought I had a stomach bug—nausea, vomiting, diarrhea. It was before we associated those symptoms with COVID," Dr. Alan said. When he first became ill, he excused himself from a medical staff meeting, and barely made it to the bathroom near his office, where he collapsed.

"I remember the cold floor as I came to. I got myself home and went to bed," he told me when I chatted with him on Zoom. The next morning he felt better and headed back to work. Later that week, he read a medical article about COVID presenting with GI symptoms, so he ordered a test. Two weeks later, the test came back positive. That was when testing was slow and before masks were routine. How many people did he and others expose in the meantime?

Nearly a year later, he's at work every day, despite his "crushing fatigue." Dr. Alan sat at his desk, framed certificates and diplomas decorate the wall behind him. Before COVID, he functioned well-above the speed limit, seven days a week. If you're old enough, you might remember the pink Energizer Bunny, a mascot for batteries who beat his drum and hopped along with boundless energy—that was Dr. Alan, but not anymore. "I work, I go home, and I go to bed. I need my sleep," he sighed, as he leaned back in his leather chair.

The trainee that gave him COVID became his patient. Dr. Alan admitted him to the hospital and discharged him five days later. Both consider themselves *long haulers*, patients with ongoing symptoms since their COVID illnesses. The trainee now fights shortness of breath. Dr. Alan struggles with ongoing weariness. Due to his personal experience and what he's seen in other survivors, he started a long hauler clinic, one of the few located in an underserved urban center.

Dr. Alan wore a crisp white dress shirt and maroon tie beneath a gray suit jacket. His beard was neatly trimmed, and the sterling gray hair that covered the nape of his neck was long enough to pull into ponytail. "I haven't cut my hair since COVID started," he said with a head bob. The pandemic left him with a different style than his shorn and clipped pre-COVID look. "But it hasn't grown here," he chuckled and pointed to his bald temples.

Employed in one of the COVID epicenters, the community is one of the most diverse in the United States. Hospital employees and physicians looked a lot like the patients, which meant they fought two wars: COVID and systemic racism. "It's too much," he said. "It's been unbelievably hard." The community is used to being on the front line of emerging global diseases. Thirty years ago, it was HIV, and then there was Zika and Ebola, among others.

In the beginning, he placed an "x" on his office calendar every day that he worked: "A hundred days straight, no breaks." There were patients to care for, medical students and residents to train and guide through the COVID craziness. "I've had 5,000 jobs and I've been in one place all my 30 years in medicine. That's unusual these days, but I love what I do. I'm making a difference in people's lives. That's what matters to me," he reported, exuding enthusiasm despite the mentions of fatigue, adding emphasis with his hands.

His passion for the mission—serving the underserved—is what drove him into medicine and kept him going day after day during the pandemic. Before COVID, he planned to work and teach until he was 99, or forever; he's rethought that after the past year. Nevertheless, he's held onto the sense of mission for himself, for his colleagues, and for the trainees.

"Some people have stepped away. I try not to judge them. I've gotten more accepting with time," he explained, crediting Dr. Wayne Jonas's book, *How Healing Works*, as a life-changing read. After reading the book about ten years ago, he made major changes: started mediating, writing in a journal, doing yoga, and eating healthier. His specialty in Family Medicine already gave him a whole person approach, but the book helped him integrate mind, body, and spirit into his life and into his approach as a healer.

Spiritual practice was an essential part of his day, even though he wasn't particularly religious. COVID demanded the spiritual grounding of Alan's palliative care and hospice work: "The hospital was never strapped to the point of deciding who got a ventilator and who didn't. But a lot of patients died, as well as some staff and a dear colleague." Dr. Alan paused for a moment, rubbing his chin, "The hardest part is the loneliness of the deaths … no family members surrounding the bed."

One of his best friends, a psychologist, fought for his life, needed a ventilator for a month, and eventually walked out of the hospital as a success story. Alan recounted that story, and admitted, "I would not have managed times like this as well in the past. I've never faced anything so challenging in my career. People who work with me say I've changed. I don't let things affect me as much. Ask my wife." (She put the Jonas book on his pillow some ten years ago, according to Alan).

Dr. Alan's ability to cope matters; many people depend on him.

With COVID came an avalanche of patients into the hospital as they tried to stop infectious exposure. At one point, the rooms and hallways of the Emergency Department had 40 patients on ventilators waiting for a hospital bed. In the worst part of the pandemic, they averaged 300 ICU patients, three times the norm, and closed outpatient clinics throughout the community to pull residents and physicians to work on the hospital wards. Some hadn't done hospital medicine for a while, but care teams were structured to give the ambulatory-focused physicians support as they relearned hospital skills. One family medicine clinic stayed open with a wellness focus, where patients refilled medications or got advice on managing chronic health issues like diabetes and high cholesterol via telehealth or in person. Another clinic took walk-ins and appointments for anyone with possible COVID symptoms. Patients were assessed, tested, and managed at the clinic, which kept them out of the Emergency Department. These changes prevented COVID exposures for staff who might have special health risks. When I spoke to him, Dr. Alan was in the process of planning the next iteration as they ramped up for distributing vaccinations.

Now almost a year since the first COVID cases, Dr. Alan's 20-hour days dwindled to 14 hours. "We are busy, doing about twice the work we did before COVID. It has slowed down since the first months, but we are working smarter and managing better. We know things we didn't in the beginning," he said.

Dr. Alan believed medicine will never be the same again and admitted human interaction has changed. "I suspect we will wear masks and avoid shaking hands for a long time." He lifted his mask off his desk and joggled it as he noted that flu cases were down as well as upper respiratory infections or "colds." "So the mask wearing and social distancing has benefited other illnesses. One of the perks of these difficult times," he said.

Dr. Alan furrowed his forehead as he told me that residents missed almost a year of their continuity clinics (where they got to know a panel of patients, following them as their primary doctor throughout the three years of residency—an essential training experience). "Some are trying to regroup and have only taken part-time jobs or are just working urgent care." Medical students studied online for almost half a year, missing important on-the-job learning in the hospital and clinics in order to be kept safe. "It will take a decade to recover. And it's shown the brokenness of US health care, the ridiculousness, the wasted dollars," he explained. Dr. Alan extolled the importance of the Right Care Alliance, which advocates for affordable and effective health care. In a system driven by profit, he said, the wealthy get too much care—over tested and over treated—and the poor are denied the most basic health care.

He feared the racism that would accompany vaccine distribution. Still, he noted, patients ask, with a brown-skinned doctor standing right in front of them, things like "When is the doctor coming?" Dr. Alan pressed his palm to his forehead and told me he hopes access to vaccines will be fair and equitable, and that his patients will accept them.

Nonetheless, he identified a silver lining: "If there is something positive in these difficult times, it is a deeper sense of team. Doctors, nurses, medical assistants, techs, transporters all pulled together. Many pushed beyond their comfort zone, to pitch in, to get the job done. A staff member received a food donation and checked to see who needed bread or lasagna. If someone wasn't doing well, they're sent home and someone else covered. We're putting our well-being at risk, but we're doing it together."

PPE was a struggle initially, but the hospital and clinics eventually secured adequate supplies. So even the transporters, orderlies or volunteers moving COVID patients from one place to another, were protected this N95 masks, face shields and gowns.

"But the rules changed," he explained. "In the past, you could be written up if you wore your N95 from one patient to the next, now the guidance is to wear the mask as long as you can, your decision. In other words, "when you sweat too much or there's too much snot, dump it."

In the past, different specialties sometimes competed and one-upped each other—the specialists were smarter than the lowly primary care doctors. In the pandemic, that stopped. Surgeons worked alongside medicine respectfully. Everyone pulled together to get the job done safely. A family medicine doctor led the ortho service to manage the COVID patients on the hospital floor, so the orthopedic surgeons could focus on surgery. Alan remarked, "In the past that was almost unthinkable. It's brought us closer. We're working more efficiently, managing twice the load and appreciating each other."

The recognition of the hard work has buoyed Dr. Alan. He heard the banging and bugling at 7 p.m. each evening. He and his team relished the appreciation the community has expressed for their "health care heroes." The experience gave him goose bumps every time. In addition, he's received emails and notes from colleagues working in other locations who are not under the same crunch: "Their support means a lot."

Some ten years ago, Dr. Alan launched a personal growth journey equipping himself to be a better person and healer. Little did he know he'd face a once in a century pandemic and assist his students, residents, colleagues and staff to address the needs of an entire community. He and his team deserve the recognition they've received.

Chapter 6 — Therese

My Story: A Lesson in Mindfulness

My sister Fran has the classic wide eyes and flat nose of Down Syndrome as well as an easy laugh and a bubbly personality. She is almost as wide as she is tall thanks to her love of food, especially hamburgers, pizza, and French fries. Severe arthritis put her in an extra-wide wheelchair in her early fifties. Dark brown curls tinged with gray frame her large brown eyes and round face, and she is quick to say, "I love you. Thanks for being my sister."

She was child number five in my family and the second with Down Syndrome. My parents bucked the times and refused to institutionalize Peter or Fran. Peter died suddenly at age six. Fran was only four years old. Some 50 years later she still remembers him fondly and talks about missing "my brother," especially when she's sad.

My parents moved her to the Sacred Heart campus's nursing home after she was hospitalized with a serious blood infection. They wanted to keep her close as they aged, and drove the few blocks from their independent-living cottage to see her several times a day. Fran and Dad read stories, played *Kings in the Corner* and other card games, as well as *Speak & Spell.* Mom monitored her menus, did her laundry, and pushed her wheelchair to the chapel for daily Mass. After my Dad died and my mother's health began to fail, we enrolled Fran in a community day-activity program so she could spend time with other special-needs peers.

When the state's first COVID-19 cases were diagnosed, the entire Sacred Heart campus shut down. Fran's sphere narrowed. No riding the van to day activities. No visits from her sisters and cousins. No visits to Assisted Living to see her mother. No arts and crafts. No sing-alongs. No chair exercises. No group meals— she ate all three alone in her room. And worst of all, no Bingo. That meant that Fran would celebrate her birthday without us.

I straddled two spheres as a physician well aware of how COVID was turning nursing homes into morgues and as a sister trying to control the care she received from 1000 miles away. I don't think being in the same city would have made much of a difference.

Birthdays had always been momentous for Fran. This year she talked about it for months before the big day. My sisters and I devised a plan to celebrate via Skype and to include Mom who lived in another building.

On Skype that day in May, I could see Fran and two of the staff wearing the glittery hats and Mardi Gras necklaces I had mailed ahead of time. One waved the still packaged banner and said, "We'll put this up in her room. But I didn't open the blow-out whistles with COVID."

I bit at my lip, should have thought of that. But Fran was focused on putting on another necklace, this one gold.

A Disney *Frozen* tablecloth covered the table. Purple plates and napkins sat next to a dozen cupcakes iced in lavender and purple that a local bakery had delivered. When Mom Skyped in, we sang *Happy Birthday*.

Fran clapped her hands and giggled, her eyes bright behind her glasses, as she basked in the attention—even though most of it radiated from a computer screen.

Mom hadn't put in her hearing aids and was befuddled as she

stared at her screen. The staff promised to deliver a cupcake to her, but it didn't reach her until the next day, a little stale.

Later I phoned Fran. "How was your party?"

"I didn't have a birthday cake," she complained.

"The cupcakes were tiny birthday cakes. What was the flavor?"

"Chocolate."

"Isn't that your favorite? What color was the icing?"

"Purple."

"Isn't that your favorite, too?"

"Yes."

"Did they taste good?"

"Yes."

"Did the nurses like them?"

"Where was the cake?" Fran was fixated and couldn't be convinced otherwise.

"We tried," I said to my sisters thinking of the effort each of us had expended. "Go have a stiff drink to the birthday celebrated without a cake and Mom without her hearing aids." I imagined a team on SNL playing out the episode; otherwise, it hurt too much.

When *Go Fund Me* campaigns began to appear for some of Fran's favorite nurse's aides who contracted COVID, it was just a matter of time. Like nursing homes everywhere, Sacred Heart covered only part of their employees' health insurance premium. Paid time off had to be earned. Many worked two jobs to make ends meet and lived with extended families.

Their situations were exactly like those of my patients in Rhode Island. At the same time, I edited my colleagues' research on stress in health care workers during the early weeks of the pandemic in Palestine. With fewer resources and poor cooperation from their occupying power, Israel, they struggled. But in the US we struggled too: poor leadership, not enough PPE, exhausted staff who were afraid and couldn't afford to take time off.

The nurse who phoned me that Friday to tell me Fran was COVID positive was one of our favorites. She knew Fran from her life before Sacred Heart. She also told me it was her last day at the facility. I held my phone against my ear and swallowed not wanting to imagine what was ahead. Over the five years that Fran lived there, we saw many come and go. Heavy loads kept the staff running and stretched thin for their entire shifts. Eventually it would become too much, and they would quit. I thanked her for caring for Fran.

"She's easy. She gives such joy."

"Will someone update us on Fran?"

"You'll get a call every day."

I sighed my relief, but that was premature.

Fran was one of the first residents at Sacred Heart to turn COVID-19 positive, so her wing transformed into the COVID area, and staff and administration struggled to implement new protocols.

Fran sounded fine on the phone, her usual husky voice, and a cartoon show blaring in the background. She functioned at the level of a second grader and complained about not having a shower, but could not tell me if she had a fever. Was her cough growing worse? She had asthma—I worried that the virus would settle into her lungs as it had in some of my patients, their oxygen levels falling and their lungs starved for breath.

No daily updates came as promised and the nurses' station never answered their phone. As her health care power of attorney, I finally texted her physician the following Monday morning.

"I'll FaceTime you when I'm in there later today," the physician typed.

Six hours later, the PPE garbed physician held her phone up to a smiling but weary Fran who waved at me. The physician lifted a sheet Fran was coloring—a bouquet of flowers in bold purple, green and pink, the marker strokes extending beyond the lines. "Look how industrious she is. Isn't this pretty," the physician said. "Don't worry. She's fine. No fever. Lungs clear."

My anxiety dissipated as I uttered my thanks.

But with COVID patients could seem fine, then crump on day five.

The facility had canceled Skype calls, but my sisters who lived nearby could visit at Fran's first floor window. Standing between the bushes and flowers, Meg read stories. Rose set up FaceTime on Fran's iPad and taught her how to use it: an aide picked up Fran's iPad and brought it to the drop-off desk. Rose then took it to her car and programmed in FaceTime. Then she sent Fran's device back inside. Standing outside Fran's window and calling Fran by phone, Rose talked her through FaceTime settings. Fran's compulsive behavior meant that she repeated tasks and phrases five or six times. It took incredible patience. I've had my own experience working with Fran and learned to count the repetitions to better manage the frustration. I told Rose that she deserved the "Most-Patient-Tech-Support-Ever" award.

Since I was conducting telehealth visits from home, I tried to make more time for Fran, taking calls and FaceTiming her several times a day. She told me what she had for lunch, and talked with my dog. We read stories that I'd picked up at the library. For the first time, I fully appreciated the unique human being she was—her easy smile and unconditional love and gratitude. She usually chirped: "Thanks for taking my call" or "Thanks for being my sister."

We counted the quarantine days left while my sisters watched Fran's laundry pile up, and worried about the cleanliness of her bathroom. Staff forgot her breakfast a few mornings. Fran complained bitterly about no showers for more than a week.

Somehow, bed-baths didn't count. Too often, she sat in wet or stool-filled pants because staff had no time to help her to the bathroom. For the most part, Fran took it in stride, better than we did.

Staff in PPE rushed in and out, but mostly Fran was alone. If it were me, I'd have climbed out the window. However, when I asked Fran how she was doing, she replied in her usual upbeat and husky voice, "Relaxing and taking it easy." And she'd show me the Word Search puzzle she was working on. I marveled at Fran's tolerance, her joyfulness despite the chaos that surrounded her.

We called and emailed nursing about the laundry, lack of shower, missed breakfasts, and a multitude of other concerns. When there was no action, Rose met with administrators—outside, socially distanced, and wearing masks. She secured cell-phone numbers.

Finally, I filed a complaint with the state health department about Fran's care and learned I was not the first to do so. Nursing homes around the US struggled to implement the changing COVID protocols, retain the staff they had, and secure temporary workers, while they tried unsuccessfully to keep COVID out. But this was my sister, our sister.

She'd attended Montessori school as a youngster and learned to read and do math. Her "taking it easy" included *The Price is Right* at 11 a.m. and *Ellen* at 4 p.m. Between her meals she read *Nancy Drew* and *People* Magazine and made dozens of calls to family and cousins. There were bundles of mail to open and cards to write. And she took "catnaps."

When I showed her my sleepy dog on FaceTime, we laughed at whether or not dogs took catnaps, too. Rarely did she admit boredom. She was a lesson in mindfulness.

She was quick to say, "You are my favorite sister." It thrilled me, even though she said the same to all of us. Her guilelessness captured the affection of the nursing home staff who pre-COVID had hidden in her room on breaks to watch television with her, or used her plugs to charge their cell phones. They, too, had fallen for "You are my favorite." But no one lingered now.

As the days mounted in quarantine, Fran started saying, "I'm lonely," and that she was missing her brother.

When Fran was symptom-free for 14 days, they moved her off the COVID-19 unit. After five years in the same room, this was potentially wrenching because Fran was compulsive about her stuff: every stuffed animal, coloring book, comb, box with her rings, and case with her necklaces had its place. Weary staff rallied to support her as she had captured their hearts.

We began securing a new living arrangement for Fran. With Mom's failing health and the COVID lockdown, Sacred Heart no longer served her needs. When we moved her out a month later, many staff ignored social distancing and hugged her. Fran tried to manage her mask as she choked up and wished her many friends goodbye.

Fran has taught me things, important things. If I slow down. If I pay attention. If I am mindful enough.

Chapter 7 — Carla

COVID Hit My Community Hard

With a smile crinkling the lines around her weary eyes, Dr. Carla said, "I'm not a hero. This is what I chose to do." She took a break from her afternoon of telehealth appointments in the Urgent Care clinic that serves much of the Spanish-speaking population in the urban center.

Carla's community fared poorly with COVID. Her parents emigrated from Honduras more than 60 years ago and settled in the New York/New Jersey area. Carla stayed in the Northeast, completed medical school and residency, and met her husband, a physician, a few years ahead of her in their residency training. They are essential workers but have higher incomes than most. She represents the increasingly diverse professionals who make up this country.

"My people have high risk jobs—bus drivers, cleaners, medical assistants, store clerks, essential jobs," Carla continued, "The pay is low and if they can't work it's a big problem. People live with extended family and friends. You have to help each other out when you're living on a small salary. These realities make it very hard to follow the COVID prevention recommendations."

On lunch breaks from work, Carla walked through the neighborhood: "Some may say it's not safe, but it's my community and I feel at home. I love walking past the bodegas and the panaderias. I say hello to people and pass their homes and apartments, the tiny gardens in pots or flowers in a window box. I feel connected. It grounds me. I find a step somewhere and eat the food I packed at home. I return to the clinic re-energized ... getting fresh air and reminding myself who I serve." Carla's mahogany eyes grew earnest as she spoke. "Of course I wear my mask. I need to do what I tell patients to do."

"I want people to take care of their community, do what they should to stay healthy and keep the community healthy. It frustrates me when they don't wear masks and participate in big gatherings. They should know better. I talk to patients during their telehealth appointments, and they are out and about. I can hear cars and neighborhood noises. One was in the elevator the other day. I know people need to get the survival basics, but they're doing more than that. I get angry."

She told me, "I get it that some feel like they have to work sick, because they need the money or their boss won't let them off. The lack of insurance, the poor living and working conditions, the loss of work, there is something unfair about all of it." Her brow creased and she rubbed her temple and leaned away from the laptop in front of her. She made a fist and her voice grew more insistent: "What infuriates me is the scapegoating of immigrants and the systemic injustice for people who look like me. It's not fair."

She described a single mother who came into the respiratory tent. Outside the Urgent Care, a tent was set up during the summer where patients who might have COVID could be assessed. Telehealth clinicians could refer patients that needed to be seen to the "respiratory tent," and staff in full PPE checked temperatures, respirations, oxygen levels, and listened to lungs. Carla worked in the tent routinely. "The mom was in her late twenties and sick. She looked like she felt horrible, sweating and short of breath. Her asthma was flaring. I was worried about her," Carla said.

Carla treated her with an inhaler—medicine the patient sucks in through her mouth into her lungs to open up the airways. "When she tested positive for COVID, I told her if she didn't get better with the prednisone I was giving her, she'd have to go to the hospital."

The mom replied, "I can't. I don't have anyone to take care of my kids."

"Certainly we can think of someone who might help you. Do you have family?"

The woman's nostrils flared, a sign of her struggle for air. "No," she said, her voice husky.

Carla hoped the prednisone would help the airway swelling and make breathing easier. She pressed on, "Do you have a friend? A neighbor?"

The woman's eyes grew moist and she wiped a tear with the back of her hand as Carla brainstormed options with her. "I didn't want to scare her, but she needed to understand that she might die if she didn't go to the hospital. COVID patients can look okay, but when we check their oxygen levels are low, too low. They can go from okay to awful quickly. And she was struggling. If things didn't turn around in the next few hours, those kids wouldn't have a Mom. I wanted to say, 'I'll take care of your kids or ask one of the nurses,' but we can't do that. There aren't enough of us." Carla squinted over her mask as she recalled the encounter, catching a tear with her finger.

Dr. Carla didn't look old enough to have three teenagers of her own. Her teens were doing a hybrid of virtual and classroom learning until the state's COVID-19 cases started to climb. More recently, they have managed fairly well with online only and have a daily routine of plugging into their computers at 9 a.m. She and her husband have created enough flexibility in their schedules to ensure that the kids keep up with their work.

"Our immediate family is spending a lot more time together. The kids miss their friends, and we don't want to expose my parents or the in-laws, so we've increased nuclear family time. We play games and watch movies, stream on television and electronic devices like everybody else. I am cooking more—I'm a good cook. We focus on eating healthy food. But it's hard to all be home together, all the time, even though our home is bigger than the homes of most of my patients. We find ways to spread out and be apart," she said.

Carla's teens binged on *The Office*, while she preferred crime dramas and listened to podcasts: "We all need escapes, to check out, to be entertained."

Carla realized long before COVID that she needed to balance the demands of work and parenting. Fifteen years of full-time primary care was burning her out; her patients had complicated health problems and lives, and so many needs: "Many were just trying to survive, thriving was a huge stretch. It's an exhausting population to care for." She switched to urgent care where she wasn't managing chronic problems day after day, week after week, month after month, and she could focus on the urgent issues. But like the single mother with COVID who was short of breath and sick enough to need hospitalization, the urgent issues weren't always easily fixable. Physicians don't learn how to find childcare for sick mothers who have no support. These are problems that need to be addressed by society. They cannot be fixed within health care.

COVID magnified the problems of poverty such as inadequate housing, unfair wages with limited benefits, underfunded schools, and insufficient social supports. The difficult life challenges of Carla's patients and her community are not easily repaired. Brown and black people can walk faster, pedal harder, run farther, scrape and pinch pennies and it makes no difference.

Drained by the pandemic, the emotional cost of witnessing the struggle of her community pushed Carla to pursue a goal she considered earlier, but put on hold—a subspecialty in Obesity Medicine. She hadn't taken the time earlier to do the course work. "Obesity has hit my community hard. I think I can make a difference. This was the silver lining of COVID for me. I got focused and completed the requirements."

Because of her own health issues, she tried to stay healthy and manage her stress. She noticed the increased stress among her coworkers—one nurse with more migraines, another suffering from frequent episodes of anxiety: "This is a tough time. We support each other. We check in. We help each other out. We find a reason to laugh. We want to take care of our patients, but we can't put our own lives, the lives of our kids at risk."

Numerous articles in medical journals, blogs, and lay magazines have examined the toll the pandemic has taken on health care workers. The well-publicized suicide of an emergency physician in New York City in April 2020, reminded of the limits of health care heroes.

Carla knew she needed to take care of herself and model that for others. She trained as a yoga teacher and attended a retreat just before COVID hit. Carla and her husband connected with some of their college, medical school, and residency friends: "We now have a routine of checking in, giving each other pep talks, and sharing jokes—it's imperative to laugh. I've been sending care packages to friends. Everyone needs a little pick me up. To know they're special."

Carla taught *Doctoring*, interviewing and physical exam skills, to first year medical students at the school she attended. She's facilitated a small group of eight students every year since her children have needed her less: "It's a way to give back. And I love it. But this year, it's hard. What a horrible time to launch a career. Learning to use the equipment is challenging enough, let alone fitting it in between the mask and face shield. You put your stethoscope in your ears to listen to a heart or lungs and it gets caught on your mask, or your earring falls out. You come in close to look in a patient's ear with the otoscope, you're wearing gloves and your fingers get sweaty because you're anxious, and then the face shield fogs with your breath. I feel for them."

The doctoring class met once a week, the only in-person class the students had, the only opportunity to create something more than a Zoom community. "But we can't bring in treats, can't have the usual end-of-the-semester party," Carla admonished. In addition, due to the worries of COVID, some clinics didn't allow their physicians to have students follow them while seeing patients, and many visits are telehealth—Carla pulled at her mask and added, "How much can you learn watching someone talk on the phone. You can't practice exam skills. Students worry that they aren't getting enough experience. It's all such a shame."

Dr. Carla resisted calling herself a hero, because she does work that she is committed to and values as a caretaker and nurturer. She knows that each of us has limits to our ability to give. The pandemic has and will continue to claim and damage the lives of COVID patients and their caregivers. Structural inequities in the US and the world cause worse loss and harm for people of color.

Carla was exasperated by the poor national leadership and the explosion of fake news. She described her own experience: "I posted a true story on Facebook about a pediatric patient I saw who tested negative for flu and had all the symptoms of COVID, but it was the point where we didn't have enough tests, so we couldn't do the test on kids. Of course, I didn't mention the patient's name. My point was the inept planning of the federal government and not enough test kits. Someone picked

it up and labelled it 'fake news.' But it was true, absolutely true."
Carla concluded with a sigh and steepled her fingers: "It has to
get better. I can't imagine it getting it much worse."

Chapter 8 — Miguel

Little Sacrifices for the Greater Good

Dr. Miguel slips seamlessly between English and Spanish. He has lived in the US his entire life, but his parents moved back to a small Mexican town 15 years ago. Spanish is the chosen language of more than half of the patients in his clinic in the Southwestern US. His dark-brown eyes exude sincerity and he speaks with a quiet confidence and competence, the kind of physician you'd be happy to identify as your own. Before COVID, he and his wife accepted two Chief Resident roles in their Family Medicine residency, two leadership positions to last one year after completing the three-year training program. "What a year it has been," he said with a head shake.

Not only were they responsible for planning the schedules, covering clinics, and fulfilling rotations in the hospital or other specialty services like cardiology and emergency, arranging vacation coverage. Suddenly they were struggling alongside faculty to keep up with the changing CDC guidelines for COVID-19. "We have a living web-based document that we constantly update every time new guidance comes out. Then we send weekly emails with updates to the teams," Miguel said. COVID also meant finding coverage for residents who needed to take off work due to COVID exposure. "We don't want people to work sick," and if exposed, initially doctors needed to quarantine for 14 days: "It's a 24/7 job."

With an MBA degree, in addition to his MD, and an interest in medical administration at some future point, Miguel is immersed in management. Change and crises have been the norm. "Before making any wide systemic changes, we needed to get the resident perspective," he told me. "Without buy-in, there's either resistance or misunderstanding. The residents have different ideas, and they need to be aired. Then my wife and I help to build consensus among them. We are much stronger when we talk with hospital administration if we have a united voice."

Several training clinics were canceled, as were some procedures—pap smears, removing moles, and cyst excisions. Time sensitive items like joint injections and circumcisions were continued. He and his wife weren't concerned, but some of the younger residents worried whether or not they'd learn everything they needed to be competent family physicians. As chief residents, Miguel and his wife were called into action and one of their first tasks was to make the clinic safe.

Prescreening protocols were created and implemented at the clinic to identify patients with possible COVID symptoms so they could be directed to locations that had enough PPE. Patients seen in person were those who absolutely had to be, and that meant creating protocols: "We tried to evaluate rashes and skin problems with video calls, but some patients didn't have the capability for that at home. We wanted to care for our own patients and keep them out of the Emergency Department if we could. Then there were our high-risk patients, such as prenatal care, patients with mental health or substance abuse issues. We didn't want them to fall through the cracks."

The next challenge was mastering telehealth. That was new to the physicians and the patients. As Miguel mastered it, he created modules to help the residents learn and presented at one of the didactic sessions. These sessions typically occurred in person on Wednesday afternoons and covered educational curricula over the three-years of residency training. Now everything was virtual. "More Zoom!!" Miguel shouted with a grin, and clapped his hands, telling me about his own challenges in mastering the "steep learning curve of telehealth." At first, it was hard to manage a patient's emotions over the phone. He admitted, "I couldn't hand the patient a tissue, or touch an arm. I learned to pause, to use silence. Sometimes it's hard to hear, and I had to figure out how to review medications and compliance when I didn't have the pill bottles sitting in front of me. I had to keep asking—how often are you taking that pill? How many do you have left? At times, I wondered how much I was really helping the patient." Dr. Miguel paused, and adjusted his dark-rimmed glasses: "I was surprised; it did get easier." He conveyed those tips to the residents and encouraged them to "be patient and sit with their initial discomfort."

Social distancing, Zooming didactics, and limiting numbers of people gathering in the clinic created isolation. To address residents' complaints of loneliness, Dr. Miguel helped to implement virtual Grand Rounds. Grand Rounds typically occurred every month for an hour in a conference room over lunch. A featured speaker gave a talk on an important topic or presented a case, then led the discussion. "With COVID, we'd canceled Grand Rounds for several month. In the new world, lunch was out, gathering together in a conference room was out, so we all mastered Zoom," he said, clapping his hands again and chuckling. He told me his wife got the idea of taking a screen shot of all the Grand Rounds attendees Zooming-in and posted it on the residency's Facebook page. "Now everyone expects to see it and it's helped with recruitment for next year's interns."

Every fall, the residency started interviewing for their next class of residents. In the past, interviews happened in person, but not this year, so the challenge was to help residents get to know the program if they hadn't experienced it as a medical student on a clinical or hospital rotation. "We tried to be creative, one of the popular events, another one of my wife's ideas, was a virtual happy hour every week for all the candidates who interviewed." His affection for his wife was obvious as he lavished her with compliments. They've worked hard to get faculty and residents to show up, as well as some of the other important team members like the social workers and nurses, "so the candidates get a feel of how terrific our residency family is."

Initially, residency faculty protected residents from managing COVID patients in the hospital. Labor and Delivery (L&D) was the first department that allowed residents to work with COVID positive or exposed patients, and Dr. Miguel led the way. He spent at least a day each week in L&D triaging and delivering babies. The intimate and supportive family environment of welcoming a new baby into the world is gone. Nurses and the doctor wear full PPE. The laboring mother breaths, sweats, and pants behind her mask. She can choose one family member to join her who commits to stay for the entire time, which may be hours. "It's an easy decision if she has a willing partner," Miguel said. "And not so easy if she's choosing between friends and parents." Mothers still breastfeed and the baby can stay with mom, but everyone is tested and monitored for COVID.

"Flexibility," Miguel said with a smirk, "The new F-word. But there are benefits." Because of telehealth, Dr. Miguel was able to care for patients who saw him at another clinic earlier in his residency. It was too far to drive or bus the distance to his new clinic site, but with telehealth he could take care of them. He said, "They were delighted to have me as their doctor again. That made me feel good. I missed them, worried about them, and they said they missed me." His whole face beamed with pride.

Another perk was working from home. He conducted administrative work and virtual teaching from his desk at home: "I can drink my drip coffee, better than the stuff in clinic, and my dogs love having me around." Frijol (bean) and Arroz (rice), each weighing in at 12 pounds or so, were the perfect size for Miguel's lap. Frijol, the older one, usually got first dibs. The other was never far from Miguel's feet.

One of Miguel's biggest challenges was personal. He couldn't celebrate his mother's birthday when she came to town. Usually she cooked for a day or more making a feast for her large family and relatives. Too many people would come to the party, and his mother arrived on a packed plane from Mexico. When his brother sent a picture of her disembarking with her mask down, Miguel freaked. She lived in a rural community in Mexico where COVID was not much of a problem. He wasn't sure how to help her understand the realities in his urban area, or how to say no to her delicious cooking, made with such love. He didn't want to offend her. "We have to make little sacrifices," he said. "I talked it over with her and tried to explain. She was disappointed, but I did see her for a meal outdoors, socially distanced and just a few people. It wasn't the same, but at least I got to see her. I told her to make sure to wear a mask, because if she brought COVID back to her small town, it could explode in terms of the number of cases. It would be awful. And the medical care is very different. Luckily, she stayed healthy. There will be next year."

The key to Miguel's coping was his personal and professional relationship with his wife. They met in college, supported each other during medical school and residency, and have shared Chief Resident roles. They bolstered each other through the pandemic, talking, venting, crying, and at times observing silence. When not on call, they came home, changed their clothes, and pulled on their walking shoes. Even before they said "walk" Frijol and

Arroz tilted their heads and raised their ears. The two mutts, part Papillon and something more, started dancing until dressed in their harnesses. "Getting outside clears our heads and the dogs love it."

Both pups were rescues, joining the household several years apart, and initially were not fond of each other. Now they pair like beans and rice.

The four-leggeds moved quickly on their short legs for long or short distances. Then Miguel and his wife shared the kitchen and cooked dinner together. If they were really exhausted, they ordered out: "Television is a great way to turn off our minds, especially comedy." His favorite show is *The Office* and he'd watched all nine seasons twelve times! "People think I'm crazy," he chortled, "but it's been a great diversion."

He and his wife sat close, their arms draped around the other. "The physical connection and hugs are so important," he said. "I can't imagine not having someone to hug in this socially distanced world." Skin is one of the five sense organs, along with sight, hearing, smell, and taste. Touch is a basic human need.

Frijol and Arroz also knew about touch and the comfort it brought, snuggling and burrowing in close. Miguel said, "They give us love, and are always next to us whether times are good or bad. They've been vital in helping us stay strong and positive during these challenging times... don't know what we'd do without our furry pals."

Chapter 9 — Reed

Sir, You Need a Mask

Reed worked in sales and marketing in the bicycle industry for thirty years. He knew the biz, in fact, probably knew a bit too much and grew impatient with the poor management in the small store where he now helped out. He'd purchased stock and set up displays for dozens of stores across the Western US. He racked up thousands of frequent flier miles to China overseeing manufacturing orders, and set up exhibits at bike shows around the world. He chuckled as he described his "spectacularly unsuccessful career in bike racing," and fondly recalled races in Northern Italy where he powered up mountains at the back of the pack. There he learned about the fine taste of vanilla ice cream and strawberries drizzled with balsamic vinegar, and of course, the Italian red wines sipped while gazing at the sun setting behind the mountains, the sky flaming with color.

In retirement, his goal was to turn wrenches and savor the simple pleasure of a project with a beginning and end, a problem diagnosed and solved. He never anticipated being an essential worker in a pandemic.

As COVID dragged on, bicycles became the new toilet paper, and at the store it was all hands on deck. Reed could do sales, but it was never his favorite part of the job—dealing with the whiny and demanding customer who is always right. With COVID, customers were frustrated, searching for ways to get active outside and entertain their stay-at-home, video-game-addicted, online-school-bleary kids. Bikes were in demand—new and used. And customers brought in old bikes for repair that had seen better days, way better days.

The shop sat between an upscale and a blue-collar neighborhood. Some customers willingly dropped hundreds of dollars or more on bike repairs without a blink; others pinched pennies.

Deemed an essential service, the bike store opened up after the initial COVID shutdown with new rules to negotiate. Mandatory masks for staff and customers. Only a certain number of customers permitted in the store at a time depending on the size of the building. Customers were to make appointments online, but who followed directions when stressed? When waiting inside the store or outside, customers were to stand six-feet apart on the patches affixed to the cement marking the distance. Bottles of hand cleaner sat near the registers, more clutter on the counter already filled with possible last minute purchases. The shop tried to be helpful by putting out signage about mask wearing and social distancing, provided masks for customers and staff, and offered training videos with the new regulations. No one wanted to enrage health department officials with noncompliance. Staff were happy to be working despite the new rules, regimen and worry. Existing only on his social security check left Reed little extra spending money for his photography hobby. During the first week, the phones rang nonstop, and there weren't enough staff people to manage the phones as customers waited inside and outside the store.

Over the summer, bikes were flying off the sales floor as if there was a "going out of business sale." Several staff spent all their time assembling new bikes and could hardly keep up. Soon stock in the supplier's warehouses began to dwindle. Parts needed for repairs, like chains, tires and tubes, became hard or impossible to find. The store started a bike "donor" pile—old bikes donated or abandoned by customers who learned the bike they'd brought from the basement or garage was too expensive to repair, or the parts were no longer available. Staff stripped the bikes for parts as needed. Brakes, gears, seat, handlebars, derailleurs—everything was fair game.

Gradually staff adjusted to the new norm, but it was a rocky, uphill grind, and customers always expected more. An avid thirty-year-old rider brought the road bike he rode every day in for repair: "When can it be ready?"

"Six weeks," Reed said, trying to maintain his "the-customer-is-first" expression despite the mask covering his lower face—a genuine, "I want to help you."

"But it's only a tune-up." Thirty looked at his bike and shook his head. "It's just routine. I bring it in at the start of every summer. What's different about this year?"

"Everything." Reeds hands flew up, palms open; he couldn't help himself. "We are six weeks out for all tune-ups. I'm sorry."

"But that's half way through summer." Thirty's face grew red and his forehead creased.

"I know and really, I'm sorry."

"I'll check somewhere else." Thirty picked up his bike and stomped out.

Good luck with that, Reed said under his breath. It's the same or worse at every shop.

The warehouses began running out of new bikes. Customers complained.

"Talk to the President about his tariffs on Chinese goods," one staffer said after an angry customer cussed at him and tromped out of the store.

Patience eroded. Biking was good for you, outside, and in the sunshine. Public Health encouraged people to go outdoors.

Restaurants created serving areas on the sidewalk. Why was this so hard? Why couldn't the store manage the need? Where were the bicycles? Customers stared at the empty floor and displays. This was a huge opportunity. Business could be booming if only there was enough stock, but there was no way anyone could have predicted or anticipated this crisis.

Customers started bringing in very old bikes for repair, bikes that looked like they'd been in the garage for a few years, or worse yet outside, next to the cabin, or maybe even the bottom of a lake—corroded frames and cracked tires. Some customers even admitted to finding them in trash bins or abandoned on the street.

One summer afternoon, a twenty-something dad in jeans and a t-shirt climbed out of his pick-up truck with a six-year old. His truck was not high end, but not a dump—no rust, tires in good condition, and no bumper stickers. He hadn't made an online appointment and slipped in behind a customer who had. He wasn't wearing a mask.

"Sir, you need a mask," Reed said.

"The virus is a hoax. It's no worse than the flu," Twenty said, his son with a cowlick and hands stuffed in his jeans pockets, tagged close behind.

"Sir, there are rules if we are going to help you."

"I just want a bike for Joe here." He turned to Joe who looked up with a pleading expression, smiling expectantly.

"Sir, we can't help you if you don't wear a mask. I have them here on the table for you to wear."

"Not wearing one," Twenty said and planted his palms on his hips, his work boots spread two feet apart.

Reed imagined him in line at the local hunting and fishing store, a mile away, either buying or selling his guns. "I'm sorry. One of our staff has a wife who is a doctor working in the ICU.

This is no hoax. This is serious."

Twenty set his jaw and stood a little more erect. "See my kid here. Joe needs a bike."

Reed didn't want this to turn into an altercation. He didn't want to be the source of a customer complaint. Luckily, the store manager had come to see what the trouble was. Reed glanced toward him. The manager shrugged his shoulders and tilted his head, a sign to serve Dad and Joe but get them out of the store.

"Well, sir, you can see our boys' bikes up there toward the front." Reed pointed. "But let's walk outside. You can see them easier through the window." Reed adjusted his mask and ushered them out the door.

This guy's belligerence grated; this was exactly why Reed only wanted to turn wrenches—who needed this type of aggravation or potential exposure? Reed was over 65, already in a high-risk group. But because they were swamped, he'd been pulled into assisting customers. If they stood out front and looked through the window, they'd minimize the indoor virus spread. He didn't bother mentioning that the manager's wife, a school teacher, was home isolating with COVID; the college age son, a diabetic on insulin, fighting COVID as well. Did the wife bring it home or the son? Who knows, but this virus was no laughing matter. But Reed knew he was wasting his breath to try and convince Joe's dad of that.

Through the front window, Reed pointed out a shiny blue boy's Trek Prccaliber, keeping his own distance from the pair as they moved in to look.

"How much?"

"$250. It's a nice bike."

Joe gazed at the bike, dragging his gym shoe across the cement, then wistfully regarded his dad.

"That's a lot. Do you have anything used?"

Now Joe eyed Reed.

"I can check. Wait here." Reed went back inside and checked the storeroom, the supply growing smaller by the hour. They'd secured used bikes from the trade-ins. Fortunately, they still had a few Joe's size. He hauled one back outside where Joe and his dad were kicking stones back and forth in the parking lot. "Bikes that fit Joe are about $150," Reed said. "What do you think of this one?"

As dad shook his head, Joe's face shifted from hopeful to glum. "Too much for us. I guess I'll try Walmart."

"Good luck." Reed said, and refrained from saying that an earlier customer had complained that Walmart and Target were both out of bikes when he'd checked.

Back in the store, Reed went straight to the hand sanitizer. He ignored the ring of the phone, put the used bike back in the storeroom, and then checked off the next customer on the list: "How can I help you?"

Impatient and irate customers' frustrations with the new world often felt directed at Reed and the other bike shop staff. Who enjoyed being a punching bag? "Some customers needed to blame someone," Reed told me. Life as they knew it had changed. The old certainties were no longer certain.

Essential workers were often targets of frustration and anger. While Reed's shop manager did a decent job of implementing the COVID safety guidelines, controlling customers and their responses was impossible. Frontline workers bore that burden, their safety at risk. We only need to watch the news to know that many have died from COVID.

Reed was not alone in being frustrated about the public's noncompliance, but Reed took care of himself by wearing a mask and cleaning his hands, staying sane by getting outside to bike, kayak, walk, take photos. Nature's cycle of buds, brilliant blossoms, blazing autumn colors, and then dormancy, marches on despite the pandemic. Reed was eloquent about being outside: "It grounds me. I start walking, pay attention to what is around me. I see ideas for photos. After awhile my body feels a little lighter. I notice the smells around me. I am in the moment. During COVID, I've gotten into a daily walking habit. That's a good thing, a necessary thing."

Chapter 10 — Jackie

Time for Common Sense

Dedicated to her patients and her community, Dr. Jackie embodies the essence of a true primary care physician. She practices in the rural south, about an hour from the town where she grew up and the residency where she trained. The largely poor, Black region suffered with COVID. The state's COVID response became a political football. "We don't have all the resources or staff we need to manage the pandemic," Jackie told me when I interviewed her on FaceTime. "But we do our best." Her voice was earnest with a note of weariness.

Medicaid was not expanded under the Affordable Care Act to include the working poor, so many patients don't have health insurance and are self-pay. In addition, Dr. Jackie's clinic didn't have the federal designation to qualify for additional staff and resources to address the many social needs of her patients. These are often referred to as social determinants of health: problems that have to be addressed to keep someone healthy, such as enough food, adequate housing, access to electricity, a refrigerator that works, etc. There is no local social worker to call when a patient needed help with groceries or securing assistance to pay their electric bills. It's all up to Jackie, her physician partner, and their nurses.

"Unfortunately, with COVID," Jackie complained, "All the attention is on the hospitals and emergency departments.

Granted they are working very hard, but primary care is kind of forgotten. Not only am I dealing with how to help my patients prevent COVID, but I also have to keep managing their diabetes, hypertension, kidney disease, obesity, and all the chronic problems that I've managed over the years. Those illnesses put them at greater risk for COVID, so we can't ignore them just because we're all worried about COVID. And don't forget the emotional relationships I have with patients. I've heard stories about their kids and grandkids. I often take care of the whole family. I'm attached. And when they're sick, I worry. When they die, it's a loss. I have to stop for a few moments at least."

Jackie summarized the challenge for primary care during the pandemic. Patients' needs related to their chronic health issues never stopped with COVID, and weren't easy to address on the phone. Dr. Jackie's patients needed and wanted to be seen by someone they knew and trusted. That put the physicians and staff at risk for infection because the patients they saw had higher rates of COVID in their communities, and sometimes they didn't know they had it. Finally, there was the emotional toll. Doctors weren't machines—they cared, they had relationships, which was imperative for healing but came with a personal cost.

Like many rural health clinics and hospitals, Jackie's was already stretched. With COVID facilities were strained further and poorly resourced with COVID tests, PPE, and staffing. The economic viability of her clinic was not at risk because it was part of a larger system. However, many primary care practices closed due to COVID. As of Fall 2020, national studies showed eight percent of practices shut their doors, around 16,000 outpatient clinics, mostly due to financial strain. That means patients without clinics located conveniently near to where they live may skip preventive care and delay the management of their chronic diseases like diabetes and heart failure. Not getting needed care puts patients at higher risk to become very sick when they contract COVID.

The decline in available primary care physicians does not bode well for the future of US health care. Primary care is about prevention and keeping chronic physical and mental health problems from needing emergency or hospital care. When it is unavailable, patients get sicker and require more expensive care and procedures. Quality suffers and costs rise. In the US we already spend more money on health care than any other country and our outcomes are much worse.

During the worst of the pandemic, hospital beds were limited. Jackie's patients didn't want to travel an hour to a bigger facility. Some didn't have the money for gas. Others wanted to stay local where their family could visit them and they knew the nurses and doctors taking care of them.

"I had a patient who failed oral antibiotics for a dental infection," Jackie told me. "The only bed was an ICU bed." The patient, who needed intravenous antibiotics, didn't really need that level of care. After much discussion with the patient and her daughter, the daughter agreed to make the hour drive. Then that evening, the daughter called Jackie.

"The sore opened up in Mom's mouth. Lots of bad tasting stuff."

"It sounds like the abscess drained," Dr. Jackie said. "How is she feeling?"

"Do we still need to make the trip to the other hospital? Can't somebody here check her?"

"Well, I was worried. I didn't want the infection to get into her blood. That's why I wanted to admit her."

"Can I just take her to the ER? It's so much easier."

Dr. Jackie sent the patient to the local Emergency Department and called to let the covering doctor know. That doctor ended up putting the patient on another oral antibiotic. "It all worked out fine," Jackie told me, "But I'm convinced that the patient lanced her own jaw abscess to avoid the hospital stay." She cocked her head to the right and rolled her eyes.

Telemedicine is a great idea, but many patients in the region don't have the internet service to support fancy video equipment. About 25 percent of citizens in the state didn't have internet, a high proportion of those living in Jackie's community, and cell service was unreliable.

"Most of the time, we can talk on the phone, but when a patient with high blood pressure and diabetes tells me they are fine, and I look at their medical chart and see they've been not so fine for the last two years—elevated blood pressure readings and high HGBA1C (blood sugar) levels, I have to see them. I tell them to come into clinic so we can check the blood pressure and poke a finger."

The clinic, located on the second floor in the outpatient wing of the local hospital, erected an outside tent so that a nurse could run downstairs and swab a patient with COVID symptoms: "But we have to have a nurse free to do that. When one or two nurses are out because they need to quarantine, that's a problem. The larger clinic in the city can send help for a half a day, but the fill-in doesn't know our routines, doesn't know where things are. So even if they are willing to make the hour drive to help us out, sometimes it doesn't help that much."

In addition, Dr. Jackie or her physician partner, who has a new baby at home, may sit with a patient for 20 minutes talking about the patient's cholesterol, high blood pressure, or another problem: "Suddenly, we realize the patient has a cough and we swab them for COVID. If they turn up positive, we've been exposed. We wear masks, but that's not foolproof, especially since we aren't wearing the N95 masks."

A level of fear comes from knowing that day in and day out

Jackie is exposed to COVID. She worries for herself, although she is young and healthy. Her medical partner worries for her baby and her husband. Jackie hasn't seen her parents and siblings, or her elderly grandmother, because she doesn't want to risk exposing them. She didn't go home for Thanksgiving, and at the time of our conversation, she wasn't sure about Christmas, even though she had received her first vaccine a week before Christmas.

Explaining how to stay safe was a challenge. Her large brown eyes grew intense as she talked about the need to be creative: "Patients live in small houses, with extended family." She told patients to wear masks inside, scrub down the only bathroom the best they can. She was proud of the way Black churches educated their congregations about staying safe, and said, "Their efforts have been overlooked." Her congregation went virtual but figured out how to rope off every third seat, re-do the entrance, and the exit, and the communion service in the big church so some members could worship together: "The pastor says we are reaching a larger group now than we were pre-COVID." Jackie thought Black churches had a role to play publicizing the value of the vaccine as well.

Mask wearing turned into a political issue in the US, thanks to the response of national leadership and some governors. In her state it was highly politicized: "I think the community understands that getting COVID is a higher risk among Blacks—more get sick and more get seriously sick. The mask wearing compliance seems better among Blacks than Whites. That's what I observe here, anyway. At the local Walmart and Dollar General, some folks don't wear masks. It's turned into a personal freedom statement. In clinic, we've had no problem with patients refusing to wear masks."

However, it's a small community with lots of the patients

and staff friending each other on Facebook. It was disturbing to know that Patient W with an appointment at 2 p.m. had a big birthday party two days ago and the FB post showed no one in the group of twenty wearing a mask: "Because my partner has a baby at home, I try to take the bulk of the possible COVID cases. I want to spare her the exposure."

This is emblematic of Jackie, who went the extra mile for her partner and her patients. She also spoke out when mask wearing was not mandated in the state, and the local school board voted down mandating masks in the schools, while teachers disagreed with the decision. Some of the board members had been Jackie's teachers and were family acquaintances. Her editorial in the local paper, entitled "Shame on All of You," discussed the importance of prevention. It created dialogue before the governor finally mandated masks. The fact that science, which she dedicated her life to, was questioned exasperated her. "It's so political I can't listen to the news as often as I used to." Jackie's face contorted as she concluded, "I just can't stomach it."

Initially, her district offered the option of in-person or virtual school for all students, and she routinely checked in with patients to see how they were doing: "It's a problem when a middle schooler that lives with grandma who is on dialysis chooses to attend in person. If the child brings COVID home, grandma is at serious risk. She could die." If they attended virtually, Jackie encouraged them. "Personally, I think it is hard for kids. In fact, I can't imagine how this works. This will impact this generation of kids. This is their future."

Jackie felt special concern about her sixth grade niece who didn't do well with distance learning: "It's hard to expect an eleven-year-old to sit in front of the computer and do their work if no one is monitoring them. And that wasn't happening with my niece." As a result, Jackie enrolled her in private school.

It cost money, but she was willing to do that. She said with a snicker, "It was a big switch to suddenly wear a plaid skirt and polo shirt every day and take Bible classes. But grandma was thrilled." Jackie didn't underestimate the adjustment: "Just when you start depending on your friends, to pick up and start all over is huge... And kids can be cliquish and mean at that age. I remember." Jackie showed me a picture of her niece in her uniform with a green backpack slung over her shoulder. "We talk. She has adjusted amazingly well. We are in conversation about whether or not she should continue with the private option next year. It's a better education," she mused. The smile lines that framed her eyes crinkled and I saw the pleasure she took in her niece's success.

Dr. Jackie was a role model for her niece. She also realized that as a young black physician, she was a leader. When she got her vaccine, she took a picture of "the shot" going in her arm and sent it to her Mom and cousins. "Sure, the history of Blacks as guinea pigs is real," Jackie said. "So is sterilization of black women and Johns Hopkins using Henrietta Lacks's cells. Both done without permission. But the worry and distrust has also been perpetuated by the Black community. There comes a time for common sense. That time is now. I can say, 'I look like you and I took the vaccine. You should too.'"

Her mother was worried though. "She told me I should have waited. She reads all the conspiracies shared on Facebook." It frustrated Jackie that people are so believing of fake news. Jackie knew she had a role as a scientist and a black woman to confront the misunderstandings and old worries. "Times are changing," she said.

Managing COVID is more than supporting her family and her physician partner, who has a new baby at home, while also keeping her patients and community healthy. It is imperative that she care for herself. As a young female physician in primary care, burnout is very real. Studies show that half (48%) of female physicians and half (46%) of family physicians suffer from burnout. Burnout is emotional exhaustion, depersonalization, or cynicism, and feelings of diminished personal efficacy or accomplishment in the context of the work environment.

One of the positives of COVID was that Jackie started doing a better job with self-care. She walks her dog more often. Fred, a Lhasa Apso mix, entered her life during medical school. She explained, "Fred loves to get out. I benefit too. I wear a mask all day. It's nice to breathe fresh air, although these winter days it's dark in the mornings and evenings." Jackie walked regularly at a park near her home; she was glad to be exercising more because she also allowed herself more treats—a soft serve ice cream cone from Chick Filet or a drive through McDonalds for a burger and fries. "I may pay for it later, but it gets me through," she joked.

She also confided, "Despite my efforts, there's a lot of tears and loneliness." In 2020, she had hoped to "put herself out there" and choose social situations where she might meet a future life partner/husband. With a chuckle, Jackie added, "My grandmother told me that I didn't have a husband because I didn't know how to sew. So I bought her a new sewing machine and bought myself one too." Unfortunately, COVID halted their sewing together and nixed all real live social gatherings, so Jackie's efforts to find a romantic partner were placed on hold.

Instead, Jackie reached out to old friends from medical school, from her residency, and to friends not associated with the medical field. With some, she said, "We Zoom and FaceTime, commiserate about being in medicine and on the front lines." With non-medical friends, she admitted, "It's good to chat about other things." Her pastor offered great support as well. He texted her inspirational messages, reminders about self-care, and shared

Bible verses. "That can carry me through the day," she said. And she reminded me about Fred, telling me about a picture of him stretched out next to her with his head on a book when he helped her study in medical school. "We have a long term relationship," she laughed.

Jackie's bravery and willingness to be a leader of change are grounded in her faith and her ability to see faith working in her life. She said, "Being from the South I have to talk about God with many patients. They expect it. In fact, they are usually the ones to bring it up. You can't practice in the rural south and not discuss God." Understanding a patient's belief often became instrumental in caring for them: "I tell patients, God has control, but we have common sense. We need to wear masks, social distance and use hygiene—do our part. Having faith doesn't mean that God will miraculously take the virus away."

Although Jackie didn't visit her grandmother because she didn't want to risk exposing her to COVID, they still talked by phone regularly: "Grandma hasn't yet mastered FaceTime." Jackie missed her sweet face, but loved hearing her strong and confident voice. She explained, "Grandma is deeply spiritual. We talk about God's role in relation to this disease. She reminds me, 'God has his ways.'" Jackie gets disheartened with how people can do all the right things and die from COVID. "Why do the good people die and the trouble makers survive? I call Grandma when I get discouraged. She many not understand some of the issues, but she always listens and eventually brings it back to God."

About her grandmother, a tiny and fit woman who looks twenty years younger than she is, Jackie said this: "She will cook Sunday dinners any day of the week, makes the best peach cobbler, and cleans her house, which is already very clean, every day." She didn't complete the eighth grade, because as one of the older children in her large family she needed to help at home.

"But Grandma is wise and she reminds me, 'God's got you and He's gonna do what He wants to do in His own time. . . And there's always a 'you just watch and see, as sho' as I tell you, it's gonna work out.'" Jackie's eyes shone as she recounted what her Grandmother said.

One of those gifts from God was a patient we'll call Mrs. V. Dr. Jackie described her as "a role model for who I want to be if I should live until 93." Mrs. V took good care of herself, was always was well groomed, and smelled good, with her hair fixed just so, her makeup neatly applied, her clothes clean and pressed. She drove herself to clinic and survived two different types of cancer. Annually, she took trips with friends, even at 93.

One morning she called the clinic and complained of a cough and loss of her senses of smell and taste, so Dr. Jackie directed her to go to the COVID tent and the nurse swabbed her. When she turned up positive, Jackie came down to talk with her. Garbed in her mask, she stood by the car where this time Mrs. V rode as a passenger; she didn't feel up to driving. "We went over the CDC guidelines and warning signs—fever, shortness of breath, chest pain, and when to come to Emergency." A week later, she was admitted to the hospital. Although, Jackie does not care for patients in the hospital, she put on PPE and visited Mrs. V in her hospital room. "That's part of primary care," Jackie said, "I care about my patients."

Mrs. V was thrilled with the young, black female hospitalist who cared for her. "You remind me of each other," she told Jackie. "You should get to know each other."

Jackie took Mrs. V's hand and said, "I promise I will."

After they prayed, Ms. V whispered, "God will take care of me."

Mrs. V recovered from the pneumonia, but the hospitalist wanted her to stay a few more days for additional respiratory therapy. "But Mrs. V needed to get home so she could vote,"

Jackie told me. "Voting was important to her. More important that a few more days in the hospital to ensure she was fully recovered."

Mrs. V voted on November 3rd and was readmitted to the hospital a few days later, and passed from COVID only days after that. After Mrs. V's death, Jackie finally connected with the hospitalist and they talked and reminisced about Mrs. V.

"She lived a long and full life," Dr. Jackie said.

"She didn't want to be intubated," the hospitalist said, "and you know what she told me?"

"God will take care of me," Jackie said.

The hospitalist smiled. "She was at peace."

Mrs. V was an inspiration to both of them, and they realized maybe they could be there for each other, two professional women of color committed to science and making sure that medicine served their community with knowledge and respect.

Chapter 11 — Irene

Ground Hog Day

Living and working near the US/Mexico border, Dr. Irene is in the heart of the COVID pandemic and the immigration crisis. In August 2020, she signed up for an early vaccine trial "to help make a difference." She told me, "People are suffering. It was something I could do. This is a terrible virus." She wasn't sure if she was in the vaccine group or the control group, but her arm was sore. A month later, she received her second shot. When she came down with a fever and chills a month later, she panicked—had COVID caught up with her? She was being so careful. With high blood pressure and carrying extra pounds, she had risk factors that can make a COVID infection serious.

Worried and exhausted, she drove to the study clinic hoping for the best. During the nasal swab, tears streamed down her cheeks as if she was sobbing. A day later, the test result was negative. She stayed home two more days until she felt better, then went back to work.

"It's like Ground Hog day! Do you remember the movie?" she asked when I chatted with her over FaceTime. The same hard work, day after day. The same routine, the same challenges. It never got any easier. Infection rates never reached a low point despite the California governor's efforts and restrictions. And the virus raged on.

Ten years ago, Irene followed love to southern California and worked in a clinic that served many low-income patients without insurance. COVID infected many of her patients and clinic staff. A third of the staff lived in Mexico, wanting affordable living and to be close to extended family and spouses without visas to enter the US.

As a family physician, one of the joys is getting to know your patients. Irene had special relationships with many of her patients cultivated over the years. Some did little things to thank her for her caring: a plate of tamales, a loaf of freshly baked bread, or a hand-painted Christmas ornament. One of Irene's favorite patients was the Christmas tree man.

Pablo was in his seventies and worked as a guard at a tree farm not far from the city. Every Christmas season he cut two fir trees and hauled them to the clinic for Dr. Irene and his nephrologist. He tied the tree to the top of her SUV in the parking lot while she worked. One year, Irene and her family picked up the tree at his home in the city's barrio neighborhood: "We met his entire family, some I already knew because they're patients. They loaded us up with fresh eggs from their chickens." The fresh pine scent filled Irene's house for the season. "I'd walk in the front door and it was like walking into a pine forest," she remembered, closing her eyes. She inhaled and said, "I am pretending to smell it." Year after year this was his gift to the doctor he trusted.

Unfortunately, Pablo contracted COVID. For the first five days, his symptoms were mild and then as with many COVID infections, he took a sudden turn for the worse. When he had trouble breathing, he was hospitalized and put on a ventilator to help him breathe, pushing oxygen into his lungs. Then his kidneys slowed down and weren't pumping the toxins out of his body, so he was hooked up to a dialysis machine to filter the poisons from the blood. Nothing worked.

Irene learned from her colleague covering the hospital service that Pablo died.

"And I didn't get to tell the Christmas tree man goodbye," Irene sobbed. As she paused to collect herself, she choked out, "I hope his wife and kids were able to tell him goodbye. But with COVID..."

The infectiousness of COVID prevents most families from surrounding loved ones during the final hours of life and at the time of death. For Irene, this was another reminder of the suffering and pain the pandemic causes. As the deaths climbed during the first surge, television news showed photos of body bags piling up in freezer trucks in New York City and elsewhere. PBS shared vignettes of people whose lives were snuffed out by COVID. The victims were spouses, fathers and mothers, brothers and sisters, grandparents, aunts, uncles, coworkers, sons and daughters.

Doctors grow attached to patients after caring for them year after year. Pablo was one of those special patients for Irene. She mourned for his family and children, and for herself. Most days, she faced the increased numbers of death certificates with an aching heart, remembering fondly Senora Y and Mrs. L. "These are hard and sad times," she said.

This Christmas her family decided to make an ecological choice and purchased an artificial tree. Irene and her family didn't want to erase their fond memories of Pablo's fragrant fir tree at Christmas.

Although Irene didn't have Pablo's gift to enjoy this year, she received another big Christmas present. She learned she had received the vaccine in the trial. "You can't imagine what a relief it was. I am sure I've been exposed to COVID a hundred times. I wear a mask and face shield, wash my hands, but day after day..."

Telehealth doesn't work for everyone, especially in the neighborhood of Irene's clinic. Homeless patients often had no cellphones. A throat needed to be looked at, or labs drawn to check a hemoglobin or thyroid level. Children needed their immunizations to prevent other illnesses like measles, mumps, and rubella; viruses and bacteria that made children sick and put some in the hospital in the 1960s and 1970s. Irene sometimes saw a patient for birth control who didn't mention that she had a cough and runny nose to the staff member who screened patients before they come into clinic.

Irene's commitment to her job required a foundation of support. The husband who drew her to California had Mr. Mom qualities. A retired firefighter and gourmet cook, he oversaw the household. He no longer had to police his college-aged children through COVID, since it's just Irene and him. He made her breakfast and packed her lunches. A sandwich, carefully tucked into a Tupperware container—the ecological choice—included lettuce from his backyard garden and homegrown San Marzano toma-toes. Best of all, there was often a handwritten note that said: I love you. Staff called Mr. Mom the Italian Madre, and asked if he'd prepare their lunches too. In the evening, she came home to shish kabob cooked on the grill, couscous stuffed peppers, fresh fish that he'd caught a day earlier, or some other mouthwatering dish. Irene felt cherished.

As a former firefighter and paramedic, he knew a bit about infection, and was more than a little concerned about Irene bringing COVID home to him, and even more worried about her getting sick. He was strict about his college age kids quarantining during their summer and winter breaks. "He's a germophobe!" Her eyes widened as she described the scene.

"I don't want your dirty scrubs in this house," Mr. Mom crowed. "Yuk. Yuk. Yuk."

After a day in the trenches, being ostracized at home was no fun. "We worked out a plan," she told me. She stripped in the garage, dumped her scrubs into a plastic bag to be laundered 24 hours later (enough time for the virus to die) and headed to the shower. Irene committed to doing the laundry. Clean and shampooed, smelling like soap, she was ready to be greeted with a welcome home hug and kiss, and a glass of Chardonnay.

The next morning Irene was back at the clinic on the front lines, garbed in mask and face shield to see patients and oversee the new world of COVID in outpatient care. With more than 20 years experience as a family physician, Irene agreed to serve as the medical lead for her clinic the year before COVID arrived. She sometimes referred to her lead role as "additional headaches for the not-so-big extra bucks." With COVID, it became an intractable headache of worry with never-ending to-dos. But Irene's stamina and rarely flagging desire to care and nurture carried her through.

With eyes that smile, Irene twisted her blonde-highlighted hair up with a clip at work. She managed with *cajoles*, apologies, and a ready laugh: "I am sorry to ask, but will you…" "You do such a great job, can you help me with…" She continued to be upbeat and always grateful for the assistance, and generous with her *thank yous*, praise, and affection.

Part of Irene's success as a leader, was the team spirit she fostered and her genuine concern for her staff and colleagues. Many who worked alongside her said, "Irene really cares." This year, staff decorated her office for her birthday with silver and mauve balloons. They taped them to the ceiling so they appeared to be filled with helium. With COVID she couldn't blow out the candles on the cake, so she used a plate to fan them out. A medical records clerk pulled her aside and said, "You are the best. Please don't ever stop being clinic lead." Once again, Dr. Irene felt cherished.

Maricela, Dr. Irene's medical assistant, worked with her for nearly 10 years. Irene called her "my angel" and said that Maricela is good at intuiting what Irene needs. When Irene sews up an incision, Maricela clipped the suture, then Irene handed the pick-ups to Maricela to line up the knots. "She's my eyes," Irene laughed. "Hers are better than my fifty-year-old pair."

Irene paid for riding lessons for Maricela's pre-teen daughter at the ranch where Irene kept her own horse. "Guadalupe (Lupe) has gained such confidence and self-assurance," Irene said. There were also Christmas and birthday bonuses because "my life would be miserable without Maricela," and a medical assistant never made that much.

When Maricela developed a fever, cough and back pain in April, Irene panicked and fired off a text. "What is your COVID result?"

Maricela texted back: "Positive 8 = (."

Irene checked in with Maricela regularly: "I told her I'd meet her at the border and admit her to my colleague's hospital service, if things got bad. I had one of the medical assistants, who lives near her, deliver an oximeter." An oximeter is a small plastic clip that fastens on the end of a finger and checks oxygen levels. Luckily, Maricela was back at Dr. Irene's side in clinic two weeks later.

A story about Dr. Irene wouldn't be complete without describing her relationship with her horse. Growing up in the Midwest, Irene started riding as a youngster. When she needed an outlet from her demanding job pre-COVID, a family member suggested she find a place to ride. Irene paid a dollar to rescue Molly from becoming dog food. A thoroughbred retired from the racetrack and bred to go fast, Molly still loved to run which suited Irene just fine. At a gallop, Irene described, "The sheer joy of the air rushing across my face, and the borrowed power and speed ... nothing matters." She waxed eloquent about the scent of sage and the dry grasses along the trails, a hawk screaming as it dove into the bushes after some rodent, and coyotes barking in the distance at dusk. Occasionally, she was lucky enough to see a bobcat cross the trail.

Irene told me, "Maricela summed it up best with her birthday gift to me." It was a stemless wine glass engraved with the phrase: "Horses make me stable."

Irene was lucky to have Mr. Mom, Maricela, and Molly supporting her during this pandemic.

Chapter 12 — Maricela

My Teeth Chattered

As Dr. Irene's medical assistant or "her right hand," Maricela's story was typical of many essential workers in Southern California. Life wasn't easy, and over the last year it became much more difficult. She pulled her thick black hair into a no-nonsense ponytail that hung down her back. Her broad brown face was deadpan as she said, "I've washed my hands so often this week I discovered last month's grocery list on my left palm." When she saw that I caught the joke, her white teeth flashed with her grin. On FaceTime, I could see the off-white walls of her house with photos behind her. She turned her phone and showed me a framed photograph of her and her husband smiling into the camera, their arms around each other, as they stood on a white sandy beach. Nearby were pictures of her two children as babies, and yearly school photos. She swept her arm and said with pride, "My family is everything."

Maricela grew up in Mexico and has family living on both sides of the border. He mother cooked at one of the best Mexican breakfast and lunch cafes in southern California and had a home in the neighborhood. Maricela's husband was deported several years ago, and continued to work and reside in Mexico. At this point, Maricela and their children lived with him, crossing the border daily for work and school. The schools were better in California.

Every weekday morning, Maricela rose at 1 a.m., packed up her kids and headed to the border. It often took up to three hours to cross. The kids slept in the darkness as Maricela drove and waited in the queue of cars at the border crossing, her radio tuned to a LatinX station. When they arrived at her mother's house, everyone slept a little longer. Then Maricela or her mother made breakfast and the kids got ready for school. She dropped them off at school and headed into the clinic. That was until California schools started distance learning with COVID.

A silver lining with COVID was that crossing the border was faster, due to fewer cars. With COVID, the kids still came with Maricela and did virtual school from her mom's house, because her husband worked. Maricela's mother cooked at the restaurant, open for take-outs, so thirteen-year-old Guadalupe (Lupe) was responsible for helping her five-year-old brother sign onto the computer. Maricela said, "My sister-in-law lives next door and she's available if there is something that Lupe can't handle. Clinic lets me out at noon so I can make them lunch. Dr. Irene is really good about helping me get away on time. The kids always reward me with good appetites and hugs." Maricela's eyes gleamed with pride.

At 5 p.m., they headed back to Mexico. The children played games on her smart phone, read books, and sang along with the radio. "They are used to it. It's just what we do," she told me.

Maricela had reservations about what her kids were learning with virtual school: "Writing with your finger on the computer screen is not the same as writing with a pencil. It's hardest for my son." She printed out the worksheets and helped him with the work when she got home in the evenings. During COVID, like most moms, she had two full-time jobs. "I worry, he is less engaged. I hope this won't get him off to a bad start, make him hate school. School should be exciting at his age. Learning letters and numbers and putting words together," she sighed. "He's still young, so hopefully there's time to catch up." She felt better about Lupe. "With all the online work, she's better with the computer and has more confidence. But I feel bad how hard I have depended on her." She described her mother's *veladoras*, thick candles inside decorated glass containers, which her mother lit each evening for her grandchildren "to keep them safe during these difficult times."

When Maricela tested COVID positive in April 2020, all she could think of was her family. Would they get sick? Had she infected them? "As soon as I felt ill, I started wearing a mask at home."

Her teeth literally chattered from the chills. Her back pain was a ten out of ten, ten being the worst on the zero-to-ten pain scale. "I felt like I was run over by a train and it was hard to lift me head off my pillow." She made an appointment at her clinic in Mexico.

The Mexican clinic swabbed her nose to test for COVID in the parking lot. The doctor prescribed blood thinner, cholesterol medicine, two antibiotics, and hydroxychloroquine— medicines Dr. Irene wasn't using in California. "Irene kind of freaked," Maricela told me. "But I live in Mexico, so I did what they told me. I also checked my oxygen with the oximeter Irene sent me."

Treatment protocols were different from those recommended by the CDC at the time, which Irene followed. In reality, Mexican doctors were ahead of the US with blood thinners, but hydroxy-chloroquine was the drug America's COVID-denying president touted, later shown to be useless, and dangerous for some.

Maricela quarantined at home. Luckily, her three-room house in Mexico had one room with its own bathroom, so she isolated there. Family knocked on the bedroom door when they delivered food to her. Lupe did almost everything—cooking, cleaning laundry, watching over her brother, helping him sign on the computer for his school work, which they did from Mexico when Maricela was sick.

Maricela sniffled as she remembered, "Lupe had her own school demands. I worried a lot. I would climb into the shower and cry. I didn't want my husband or the kids to hear me."

As an essential worker in transportation, her husband wasn't allowed to take time off. "He tried to come home and check on me when he had a break. He worried so."

"And Dr. Irene worried. She woke up one night with a nightmare that I was dying and texted me, 'Are you okay???'" Maricela told me she texted Irene back: "I'm actually feeling better. Don't worry."

Miraculously, no one else in Maricela's immediate family got sick. Accolades to her for being very careful. However, she had a cousin who ended up in an ICU in Mexico. "His lungs were not doing very well so they induced a coma and put him on a ventilator. His wife can't see him and he can't talk to her. It's so hard for them. And all we can do to help is pray."

The pandemic was hardest on her son who missed his friends and didn't understand why he couldn't go to the store and help Maricela like he used to. "It's stricter here in Mexico," she said. "Kids aren't allowed in the stores, and only one person per family is allowed inside at a time."

Maricela's first day back at work was his birthday. "Celebrating his birthday was awful because we couldn't have a big party with his *tias y tios, abuelas y abuelos* like we usually do. It was just mom, dad and his sister—boring."

Maricela knew to be cautious. "I know how awful I felt with this virus. I thought I might die, I felt so bad." She did not permit her family to attend her mother-in-law's gatherings, 10 to 12 people in the home, "too many, not safe." Maricela and her children walked their dog in a nearby park at 6:30 in the evenings: "The kids and the dog need to run out their energy. Dad joins us when he can. It's quiet, not many people are out." Sometimes the kids rode their bikes. Their house has a patio where the children got outside to play during the day. "My son likes to drive his trucks over the tiles—*vroom, vroom*. He has lots of fun."

Maricela's forehead furrowed and her eyebrows angled toward the top of her nose when I asked her what kept her going. "My family," she said. "I have to keep going for my kids and my husband. Family is the treasure I have."

Maricela worried about people's emotional lives, and the fact that more adults and kids were depressed. COVID affected health and emotions. She was angered because some people didn't believe this was a pandemic. "But family keeps me going. And we have it better than many."

Chapter 13 — Therese

My Story: Giving Up the Sisyphus Role

When my Mom turned 90 at the end of May 2020, she was residing in Assisted Living on the Sacred Heart campus. We'd moved her there 10 months earlier when she broke her shoulder because of a fall. She left the independent living cottage reluctantly and adjusted slowly, but staff talked about how sweet and gracious she was, always apologizing for being a burden.

There was group exercise class, and spelling bee challenges, but bingo and old-time movies with Gene Kelly were of no interest—"for old folk." Her foot nurse came to trim her toenails. We took her out every six weeks to get her hair colored and cut, and invited her for lunch. Family and friends visited her frequently. Fran, her 57-year-old Down syndrome daughter, who lived in another building on the same campus, came to her room weekly for lunch. Mom kept a purple box with "Fran's stuff" in her room—coloring books, crayons, puzzles, and Old Maid. She treasured her role as a mother.

Shortly before COVID closed the campus, Mom pulled her college-dorm size refrigerator onto her leg when Fran was visiting. That resulted in a trip to Emergency for x-rays, followed by a check for blood clots a week later, and days and days of sitting with her leg up. Fran's visits for lunch ended, and Mom didn't forget to use her walker as often.

For her 90th celebration during the pandemic, we couldn't

enter and she wasn't allowed out, and she'd never hear family singing under her window from her third floor room. We canceled all our pre-COVID party plans and decided to order dinner at a nearby seafood restaurant, her favorite. Her old parish priest, Fr. Donald, now the chaplain at Sacred Heart, agreed to pick up the meals and join her. As a member of the staff, he was permitted to visit residents. We also sent a bottle of wine, red roses, and Prices candy, as my Dad had done in his later years.

All five daughters called and sang to Mom at various times during the day. Bundles of birthday cards and more bouquets of flowers, which perfumed her room, arrived from family and friends. Having the priest all to herself was close to heaven. Mom loved men and was still a flirt in her ninth decade. She and the priest reminisced about my father, and talked politics. The priest said, "If Orange Hair has four more years, I'm moving to Canada and I'll take you with me as my housekeeper."

Mom told and retold the punch line. We had all long since made our peace with the fact that she was a 1950s style wife and mother who lived to be appreciated by men, and that her greatest desire in life had been to be a homemaker. None of us dared to disparage the priest's sexist comment. Her independent career-minded daughters were both a joy and curse.

After the birthday, the weeks dragged. Meals alone in her room. Limited walking the halls. No visits to chapel, only Mass via the internal channel. Exercise class and the Spelling Bee canceled. Mom was lonely and bored. Her long, gray hair annoyed her, as did everything else.

Outside visits on the porch were allowed for a few weeks, but the facility never installed plexiglass for safe inside visits as recommended by the state health department. So rain canceled everything. When staff began to contract COVID, all visits stopped and family was back to standing three stories down and waving to Mom as we talked with her on her phone. We dropped off lotion, summer tops, and socks or other personal items she needed at the designated entrance for staff to deliver to her. We attempted to see her through Skype and FaceTime, trying to quell her anxiety and frustration with her prison-like environment. But she was perplexed without help, and staff had no time to assist her when we called. Photos and messages sent through email went unread. Our over-the-phone tech support had mixed success.

I asked if Mom's foot nurse could enter to trim her painful toes, because she was a nurse. Denied! Could Assisted Living hire an internal hair stylist, someone safe? Denied! I completed an application to the state Ombudsman to see if Mom qualified for the "essential caregiver accommodation," allowing one daughter to routinely visit Mom face-to-face. The representative interviewed Mom, but my calls about the outcome weren't returned.

When Mom broke a tooth, she was allowed to go to the dentist. Due to the late hour, facility transportation was not available, and Mom hated it anyway. Her daughter Rose took her, and after the appointment, they checked on the new recliner, her belated birthday present, and chose the fabric—a lovely gray blue. Mom was thrilled to be out, the truancy a balm to her spirit, despite the mask.

With the lingering experience of freedom, she begged Rose to spring her out for a haircut and color. On their way out, Rose rolled Mom over to Fran's first-floor window in the nursing home. Fran was one of the first to contract COVID on the campus, and was serving out her 14-day quarantine on the COVID ward. It was nearly five months since they'd been together in Mom's room. They waved through the glass and blew kisses.

That afternoon, I received a call from the director of nursing, "What were Rose and your mother doing near the COVID ward?"

I didn't squeal, but the fresh haircut and style made it obvious. Administration reprimanded Rose, and quarantined Mom in her room for 14 days. It felt like punishment, and she didn't really understand what she'd done wrong. Mom wanted to see her special needs daughter. We'd been asking if staff could wheel her over to see Fran at her window for months.

Whenever I called, I dialed two times in succession to give Mom enough time to get to her phone. We worried the confinement was making her weaker, and she fell again.

"I hear you have a black eye," I said, "How are you doing?"

"I'm a little sore. It's so boring here."

"I am sure it is. Are you reading?"

"Sometimes my eyes don't focus."

"Are you wearing your glasses?" Sometimes she misplaced them. We'd declined sending her to the hospital for a head CT scan with the fall. Mom wanted no more hospitalizations and we supported that. Head x-rays, where the machine came to her, had shown no broken face bones.

"Yes. I wish I could see Fran again. I worry about her."

"We're checking on Fran. She's in her new room and good with FaceTime."

"Where did you go for the weekend?"

"We stayed home, Mom. Everything is closed with Covid."

"Are you sleeping?"

"Thankfully."

"Are you allowed to go to chapel?"

"No, but I watch Mass on the campus station. Fr. Don says it. And he brings me Communion," she chuckled. "I don't think he's supposed to, but he wears a mask."

A few days later: *Chime. Chime. Chime.* My cell sounds like cathedral bells. Caller ID told me Assisted Living was calling. I clutched the phone next to my ear and inhaled. Mom was

COVID positive. I braced myself.

Her move to the COVID ward, the same building where Fran had been, yielded more grayness. Her first floor room had an outside window, so my sisters saw the effects of her fall a week earlier. The bruising around her swollen black eye extended to her jaw. She needed to pry her eyelids open with her fingers to see. She shivered in a cotton hospital gown and pullups, adult diapers.

"Can you get me my bathrobe and slippers? I was allowed to bring this." She pointed to a basket of items on the hospital-style table: iPad, cell phone, wallet, glasses. But none of her own clothes.

When I learned that administration planned to keep patients in gowns and pullups, I saw red—they expected patients who were up and moving around to wear open-backed hospital nighties and adult diapers for two weeks, 14 days!

Granted, the facility was in over their heads: increasing numbers of staff out sick and stretched thin, temporary staff trying to fill in, inexperienced managers with poor medical support for implementing the changing CDC guidelines.

Up to that point, my sisters and I had plied administration with emails and phone calls using a honey instead of vinegar tactic. That afternoon, we bought brand new clothes for mom. If administration was worried about infected personal clothing, we'd try to work with them. But when reception staff wouldn't accept them, I called the CEO's cell phone telling her voicemail how appalled I was with the institution's lack of respect for the dignity of their aging clients. The next morning, administration relented—"Our policy for admission is to change the resident into a clean gown as we also clean the room and change sheets after removing clothes—this is precautionary measures for viral shedding. Patients have the right to wear their own clothes... As you are aware we have lost staff members due to this outbreak."

Suddenly it hit me. The facility did not have the bandwidth to do better. My efforts to push Sacred Heart to be more creative about improving the quality of life, to eliminate the prison-like environment, to follow CDC guidelines was wasted breath.

Somehow, the realization made it easier. I quit struggling to roll the immense boulder up the hill like the mythical Sisyphus. I was still in the underworld, sitting next to the boulder, but moving the boulder was no longer my responsibility. And I wasn't alone. Thousands of families were facing the same predicament—watching distressed loved ones suffer and unable to intervene. And worse yet, they were prevented from comforting their loved ones, and worried they might never see them again.

Mom wore her stylish new turtlenecks and slacks, and complained about the coughing and talkative roommate who joined her on quarantine-day five. They had so many new cases that they were assigning two patients to a room. So much for my request to give Mom a single room.

After I heard the roommate hacking in the background when I checked in with Mom, I reminded the medical team that the CDC had new guidelines. Quarantine ended 10 days after first symptoms or positive test, not the previous 14 days.

"Staff is really busy, we might have to wait until Monday," the doctor told me.

I bit my tongue and clutched my cellphone in my sweaty palm.

Unexpectedly, they moved her back into her own room on day 10 and even allowed her to see Fran in the courtyard. Two COVID survivors. We were grateful and elated. She had conquered COVID—no cough, no fever, and no breathing problems.

Mom wasn't sure what all the to-do was about. She felt just fine, except that she couldn't cover up her bruised face with makeup. She was back on the third floor, where she sat miserable and alone looking down at us standing in the garden three stories below her window. We worked to retrieve her few belongings, including the most important—a photo of my Dad dressed in his navy uniform as a young officer. Her cell phone and charger never reappeared—stolen or lost in the laundry.

When I FaceTimed with Mom and watched her try to figure out how to flip her iPad so she could show me a picture someone sent her, I realized how much she had declined. It took nearly ten minutes. I asked her physician to consult hospice while my sisters and I discussed moving her to a smaller facility and explored living options with an administration committed to maintaining her dignity and quality of life. Rose toured several facilities, as much as she could tour with COVID.

A month later, after much discussion and with Mom's permission, we moved her into a smaller facility. I drove home to help with the move. It was the first time I'd seen her in person in five months. Frail and fragile, hunched in her recliner, she proudly showed me the single box she had managed to pack the day before. As my sister bellowed out tasks and I packed, my mother half-heartedly welcomed the staff coming to wish her well. The activities director, who'd restarted group exercise earlier that week, wondered if mom needed a distraction. An elderly male with a comb-over balanced on his cane and sang her a love song from the forties. Her nurse, who had confided in Mom about a difficult marriage, wept.

Due to COVID, we weren't allowed to organize her room in the new facility. Standing in the wind and sleet outside Mom's first floor window, we shouted and pointed trying to direct a staff person inside. Mom sat in her recliner dazed and overwhelmed. The falling dusk forced us to call it quits. Maybe it was just as well; maybe she'd seen enough of us that day.

The gift of the new facility was in-person, face-to-face visits. I arranged one for the next day. Garbed in face shield and mask,

I could sit in the lobby by the fireplace, or in another room with a comfortable couch and more privacy. I chose the latter and watched Mom inch toward me with her walker, the curve of her spine from scoliosis more dramatic than I remembered.

Once settled into the upholstered armchair, she began to cry. I found a box of tissues and handed her one.

"I don't like it here... I decided too fast," she cried, while mopping her face and honking into the tissue.

Winter's gloom filled the room and roiled through my chest. "I'm sorry," I said. I wasn't supposed to touch, let alone, hug her. But that was what she needed.

"This is so hard," she wept.

I searched for words, how to help her move forward. At least I was with here in person. That would never have happened in the old place. We thought she wanted to see her daughters. Or did we misread her, was she missing the familiarity of the old place and friendships we didn't know she had? "I'm so sorry. COVID is making everyone's lives miserable. I'm sorry you are going through this. You've faced many hard things in your life."

More tears. "I think I need some cash."

"What do you need to buy?"

"I'd like some."

"You can't go out with COVID. They'll put your haircut on the monthly room bill."

"It would be good to have some tens and twenties."

"You wallet's locked up at the nurses' station. You just need to ask." She had no need for money. She'd gone through several hundred dollars during lockdown at the other facility. Someone stole it, or maybe she was tipping staff. Or had she asked one of the aides to purchase items that she didn't want us to know about—incontinence pads, candy? How hard it must be to have your daughters know all your business.

"It's hard to get used to a new place," I said. "How's the food?" They supposedly had a gourmet chef.

"Awful. Cold cereal for breakfast." It would take her a week to learn that she could ask for hot oatmeal.

We waded through the gloom, crumbs of reassurance on my tongue. Ignoring the rules, I reached out and held her hand. "What do you like about your room?" The facility was constructed less than five years earlier.

"Not much."

"Mom, you've been through tough things before."

The mother of six, two with Down syndrome. The death of a child who was only six years old. Her grandchildren lived out of town. A daughter fought breast cancer in her forties; another had a stroke at age fifty. She had moxie. How did I help her find it? And could I? Did she still have access to it?

"Grit," she mumbled through her tears.

I nodded, encouraging her, wanting to hug her. My own battle churned—the helplessness of witnessing her misery and the realization that I could do nothing. As a physician, I'm used to controlling things.

"You just do it," she uttered through fresh tears.

"Yes."

I fumbled on inarticulately until staff said it was time. I managed a half-hug before the nurse walked her around the corner toward her room. I stood shaking and then plodded out to my car. I was headed back to Rhode Island the next day. Who knew when I'd see her again? At that moment, children and parents all over America were wondering the same thing as they said goodbye to their loved ones.

COVID infection rates in the county climbed, but the new facility allowed group exercise, group meals, and a safe stylist who cut hair. Mom complained, but showed off her new trim, and told me about the compliments she received regarding her lovely thick, gray hair. My sisters visited during in-person lobby appointments and outside at her window. We rode the tides of mom's objections. She didn't know anyone. There was no chapel, so god wasn't present. Too many people weren't in their right mind. She didn't fit in. It had been weeks since they'd changed her bed. She was overdue for a shower.

She complained to my sisters that I was the one who forced her to move.

"I have broad shoulders," I told them.

I tried to sort through the fact and fiction of Mom's growing confusion. Had her sheets not been changed for three weeks? But she loved exercise class, they played some game with yellow foam noodles and Jim, the twenty-something trainer, was terrific. The facility sent out a photo of their trip to see Christmas lights, with Mom seated in the facility van, wearing a set of antlers on her head with a big smile on her face.

In person visits stopped when a staff member contracted COVID just before the holidays, but family could still stand outside her window. My sister wanted to have her over for Christmas Eve, but that meant 14 days confined to her room, and she was enjoying the activities.

I explained several times about the severity of COVID, that we couldn't take her out because we didn't want her confined to her room again. However, on Christmas day she asked, "Who's picking me up?"

When the activities director turned COVID-positive and twenty residents were afflicted, mom, one of the healthy ones, was jailed in her room again.

One evening, my sister received a panicked call from Mom at a time Mom was usually in bed. "I'm looking for Bill, but I know he's dead." Bill was her husband of 62 years.

"Maybe he's calling to you?" my sister said, knowing Mom's religious beliefs.

"And I'm worried about Fran. I need to kiss her good night." Fran was her Down syndrome daughter.

"Mom, Fran's fine. She lives in the group home. You don't need to worry about her."

"I know I'm confused, but it all feels so real."

Finally, the two weeks passed, and Mom was allowed out of her room. Immunity from her previous infection had kept her safe. That evening my phone chimed. Mom had fallen and bumped her head while she was simultaneously using her key to open her door and unpeeling the foil from a chocolate kiss. I wanted to scream—what were you thinking? Haven't you learned to be more careful?

"Our policy is to send head injuries to Emergency for evaluation," the nurse said. But Mom hadn't lost consciousness and reportedly looked fine.

"My mother doesn't want further hospitalizations. We've made that very clear. Family does not consent to her going to the hospital. Please call hospice." I hung up thinking the nurse had understood.

Four hours later the Emergency Department called. The receptionist was trying to find my mother a way home so we didn't incur $500 for the transport. I bit back my fury. I am a physician, my mother's power of attorney, and my directions were ignored.

I'd been on the receiving end of nursing home patients in the Emergency Room. Crazy, especially during COVID, for the facility to expose a frail elder just to protect themselves against a lawsuit. Cover your ass medicine. Quality of life and respect for dignity ignored. Of course, x-rays and a head and neck CT were done. The for-profit health care system racked up dollars that didn't improve quality of life, but confirmed her vascular dementia.

When I checked in with her, she fretted, "I've been looking for my credit card all day."

"Mom," I tried to calm her. "It's in your wallet which is locked up at the nurses' station."

"Oh."

"Did you need it for something?"

"No, I didn't want to lose it."

I wondered if this was the brain fog that sometimes follows COVID infections, in addition to the dementia.

Now Mom wants to return to Sacred Heart. She tells me, "The people here aren't in their right minds." She also misses the chapel. Granted, her last visit to the chapel at Sacred Heart was almost a year ago as COVID shut it down long before we moved her.

With my heart bursting, I stare out the window as I type. Writing helps me make sense of these times. Winter is holding on in Rhode Island. The small geese that spend the season bob along in the rough water unbothered by the blustery wind. They wear soft black and charcoal gray tuxedos and a white bowtie circles their necks just under their black heads. Over a thousand arrive in the fall, and they gather in groups of a dozen or more riding the peaks and troughs of the waves in front of our house. Security and fortitude in numbers. Their *ruck, ruck* is a comforting sound. They call to each other at night as well. With the lengthening days, they will eventually head north to their breeding grounds in the Artic tundra. But I trust that their *ruck, ruck* will comfort me again next winter.

Chapter 14 — Susan

I Needed a Good Laugh

COVID made our public schools a rapidly changing land-scape. In Spring 2020, distance learning was suddenly introduced. Then schools in many communities straddled a hybrid version of online and in-person instruction. In the last few months there have been efforts to get students back in the classroom full-time. Susan was in the thick of it as a school nurse in a public school located in a diverse urban neighborhood. She's also the mother of four teens trying to negotiate this shifting world: twins at college, one in high school, and the youngest, an eighth-grade special needs student.

Susan, in her forties, talked with me from the desk in her "home school office." She spoke fast and chuckled every few sentences. She's someone who would probably do a few extra laps around the track when training for a race.

When all four kids were finally in school, she started her nursing studies. Together, they left home in the morning and did their homework around the kitchen table in the evenings. In between, with some support from her husband who worked full-time, she squeezed in all the tasks a mom does: meals, laundry, cleaning, parent-teacher meetings, homework help, soccer and basketball games, taxi services, and feed and walk the dog, if nobody else did.

In her first years as a new nurse, she was relegated to the

night shift at the hospital. It was taxing, and it was hard trying to manage the job and family obligations. She wasn't a twenty-something anymore and she did need to sleep a little. After several years, she took a job as a school nurse, hoping the eight to four shifts and the summers off would be easier on her and her family. She'd experienced school nurses with her own kids' school emergencies, including a bad reaction to a bee sting. Her youngest daughter received specialized help due to a visual disability. Sally's IEP (Individualized Educational Plan) provided a vision therapist who worked with her at school, which made a big difference in her ability to learn. Susan figured she'd have more flexibility as a school nurse and hoped she could make a difference in the lives of the students. Her mom taught for 30 years on Native American reservations. Watching her own mother, Susan knew what a good educational experience meant and how much physical and mental health played a part.

With special needs children mainstreamed and integrated into regular classes, school nursing is more than handing out acetaminophen for a headache, applying a bandage to a cut, and deciding if a child should go home. Now there are feeding tubes to manage, asthma action plans and inhalers, epi-pens for anaphylaxis (allergic reactions). And if families don't speak English and 80 percent of the children qualify for a free or reduced-cost lunch, a nurse needs a wide range of social service skills.

Susan was finding her stride, eight months into her school nurse position, when COVID hit.

"Actually, managing the nursing role online was like starting a brand new job," Susan told me. "The worse part was my self-worth; I couldn't help families like I wanted to. Several weeks in, I thought about going back to the hospital." She shrugged her shoulders with a sigh.

"I felt like I was working all the time and neglecting my family."

Her solution was to create a routine and schedule. Every morning she went into her office and closed the door—the room where she sat talking with me. The walls were white, and paper piles were stacked on the pale wooden table. A photograph of her family acting silly hung on the wall behind her.

She would take a break for lunch, check on the kids, and go right back to work. She closed the computer and ended her day at 4 p.m. She told me, "I'd have a glass of wine. You can't work and drink." She laughed, "Or you shouldn't. That helped me know when I was done."

COVID brought one silver lining to the school—administration finally contracted with a translation service. "Before COVID, I'd want to phone a parent about an emergency, or a child needing to go home, and I'd call around to find someone who could get on the call with the parent and me." Susan said with a scoff. "I could spend an hour or more trying to find a Spanish speaker." The families at the school spoke six different languages.

With the new language line, she talked more reliably with the parents. Tough conversations with a translator concerning the attendance of Koa or Jose still weren't easy: "I'd call and try to not offend the parent as I asked why Koa wasn't signing on. Many parents were in survival mode, and for some, school for their kid was one more complication. Eventually it would end with the parent telling me, 'I don't want your help. I'm not sending my child to school right now.'" Susan shook her head and frowned. "They were trying to stay afloat. I couldn't blame them. But…"

The school quickly realized that some pupils were falling off the map. Almost 50 needed reaching out to. Some didn't show up for the morning check-in, didn't turn in assignments, or weren't participating at all. Administration quickly formed an SOS team composed of the principal and assistant, counselor, social worker, several support staff, and Susan. These were difficult situations with big extended families, non-English speakers, living in close quarters. Many of the adults were essential workers; many contracted COVID. The social worker managed the families who needed food, housing, or support to keep the utilities on. Some issues were as simple as needing an internet hot spot or fixing an iPad. Even those requests weren't so straightforward. They required submitting a tech ticket and arranging transportation to pick up and drop off the technology. And of course, with COVID it included protective equipment and social distancing.

"I did a lot of work in the driveway with my mask on," Susan told me. She dealt with problems such as helping a child get glasses or assessing for hyperactivity. COVID made none of this easy. Securing an eye or hearing test or the diagnosis of attention deficit disorder meant faxing requests. And the school building was only open on Tuesdays and Thursdays. Susan said, "I was a faxing maniac on Tuesday, and I prayed that I'd have a whole stack of medical records sent back to me by Thursday." She laughed heartily and her smile lines crinkled, "In my dreams. Of course, some faxes didn't go through, and you know what the medical offices are like right now."

Negotiating the new landscape with all its limitations and constraints allowed the SOS team to develop trust. Together they worked through their hurdles. They figured out the most efficient way to manage the many hoops of submitting requests and making sure they were received. After completing the long list of necessary tasks, and problem solving the inevitable obstacles, they grew into a well-oiled team.

Susan paused for a breath and raked her fingers through her curly hair, "Then I needed my own personal SOS team. The 'I'm a horrible mom' feeling took hold of me. I realized my Sally was miserable with all the screen time. Tired eyes and headaches. No vision teacher to help her at home. Lots of tears."

Like the Moms across the nation, when Susan finished her own full-time job (or when she could take breaks), she worked at her other full-time job—helping her kids negotiate online school. This was earning her the "'Worst-Mom-Ever Award,' as the enforcer of all mandates."

After sitting for hours with Sally to help her with schoolwork, she finally admitted to herself that Sally was having trouble. "I kind of ignored it for a while." She was too consumed with figuring out how to do the nurse thing virtually. "I'm so embarrassed, but when I finally gave her time, I realized Sally's problem was bigger than I could manage."

Sally had undiagnosed ADHD. And her eye problem made all the screen time nearly impossible.

Her vision wasn't bad enough for Braille and audio books cost $30 apiece. "Do you know how many books they use? Thirty a pop is beyond our budget," Susan said. "And have you ever listened to the free audible apps? They're a computerized voice that sounds like Siri—guaranteed to put an insomniac to sleep." She imitated a few lines in a slow monotone voice and throws up her hands with a combined laugh and sigh.

It took a while to secure a diagnosis for ADHD for Sally by way of telemedicine and limited in-person visits, but once accomplished, things improved. Sally was also missing her friends and basketball practice. Since her dad was the eighth-grade coach at a private school, it worked for her to be on the team despite her vision issues.

Susan's humor was obviously an important survival tool. With a snicker, she described getting the every two-week COVID test for teachers implemented. Teachers needed to register online before the tests could be collected. The registration seemed simple enough. Susan sent out an email with the link for signup, and then staff would come to her office and receive a vial to spit in. This was repeated every two weeks. "The thought of driving dozens of vials of saliva to UPS for mailing wasn't on my favorite-thing-to-do list," Susan said, "but it's part of the job." As the process kicked off, she started getting emails reporting that the sign-up link wasn't working, which she ignored for a while. She was busy trying to collect medication administration permissions for the students with seizures, and action plans for her 40 asthmatics by visiting parents in driveways and cajoling the medical offices that were still overwhelmed by the new world. After the thirteenth or fourteenth complaint, Susan decided she needed to check. To her horror, the link the Department of Education (DOE) had sent opened to sexual dysfunction screening questions. The male teachers dutifully completed the form. (Maybe COVID affected erections. New information is being reported every day.) The female teachers were the ones who complained. Susan immediately informed the DOE—then she howled with laughter. "As tears streamed down my beet red face, the maintenance crew passed my office and asked if I was okay," she said and added, "I needed a good laugh. I coasted off that for the rest of the day."

Once physically back in the school building, Susan walked into an entirely different job. There were the anxious teachers who sent kids home with a sniffle, without letting Susan know. There was the teacher worried about getting the virus, but who wore a bandana for a mask. "I gave him my medical-grade mask spiel."

And now it mattered that her office didn't have a door. "How can you have an isolation room without a door?" She shook her head. "So, I went to Lowe's and bought a zipper-sealed door. The kids love the zipper as they wait inside for a parent to pick them up." When Susan had a kid in her room, she had to move out into the hall. "I now have my 'office-box', a box I throw all my paraphernalia in when I have to make a move."

"Of course there was more," she told me. The cleaning crew used a liquid spray that curled her papers, so she has to stuff the remaining papers into a drawer. "Curled papers aren't terribly professional and a little harder to get into the FAX machine." Another chuckle spilled out.

Then there was the task of ordering PPE. Administration was in charge. "But they had no idea about what was needed. We ended up with extra-large gloves only. Clearly, a man placed that order." Susan rolled her eyes, then describes a mind-numbing conversation with the administration in which she explained the importance of face shields and proper masks. "I finally said, 'There is no choice here. You can't not get them. You have to.'"

She bemoaned the utter impossibility of inventorying the needs for the entire school. At the same time she tried to get her protocols in place for doffing and donning PPE, testing, and contract tracing. Plus how to manage the autism spectrum kids and deal with the spitters and fighters who couldn't wear masks or social distance. And then there were the PPE needs outside the classroom—teacher assistants (TAs) who rode on the bus with the students, within six feet of another person for more than fifteen minutes, needed to be included in the count.

Susan had other worries. Privacy rules prohibited revealing the names of students who test COVID-positive. That raised the challenge of figuring out when a TA might be exposed to a student because TAs didn't ride the bus every day. Susan's solution: "Have the TAs keep a schedule of when they work and turn it in. But it's one more thing to attend to. Some days I think my head will explode."

Susan was in the thick of the evolving world of in-person schools operating during a pandemic. Unfortunately, many schools did not have enough staff or financial support to have nurses like Susan to sort through the morass. Susan's humor pulled her through, but she said with a laugh, "Check back in a month. I'll have more stories, and hopefully, I'll have my new routine figured out." Then she winked, "And I'll let you know how I'm doing with 'The Worst-Mom-Ever Award.'"

Conclusion

The Spanish Flu killed 50 million in 1918. Before that the bubonic plague, also known as the Black Death, ended 25 million lives. Pestilence and plague wreaked havoc and suffering in the Bible, Torah, Quran, and Gita. Overcoming drought, famine, disease, and war seems to be a recurring challenge for humanity.

COVID-19 is the great threat of our time, a new, novel virus our immune systems were not prepared to fight. Our bodies do not have cells, proteins, or chemicals that recognize COVID. At the one-year anniversary of this 21st century pandemic, the number of deaths in the United States has reached over a half million, more than the number of US soldiers killed in WWI, WWII, and Vietnam Wars combined.

As I conclude these *Chronicles,* my goal is to avoid well-worn platitudes such as "think positive" or "what doesn't kill you makes you stronger" or "things happen for a reason." Such clichés trivialize the struggle and pain these essential workers have witnessed and personally endured. The immense impact of this pandemic in suffering and loss is individual and tragic, and too often lonely, but there are losses to our families and communities, as well. These costs include almost unmeasurable social and economic impacts; many are only just being identified. These impacts have the potential to have long lasting negative effects.

Therefore, I write to find my own way forward, my own path to recovery and peace. During these interviews, I am heartened by the multitude of strategies that these essential workers have employed to survive and even thrive. I sort through and reread my journal entries as I negotiate my combined roles of doctor and daughter/sister, hoping to gain momentum and confidence. For me these people and the conversations we had were like the red, yellow, and lavender flowers popping out of the rocky and trash-strewn desert hill in Palestine—hope in a place of seemingly endless struggle and strife.

What follows are the main themes I have pulled from these stories. I encourage you to add your own.

Potentially, hope…

We have the promise of vaccines, but the realities of the broad global distribution required to bring the virus under control is a challenge. It is the same old story of "taking care of our own first," which leaves the poorest countries with some of the most vulnerable populations at the back of the line for receiving vaccines. Even with COVAX, the program run by the WHO (World Health Organization), and the pleading of the Secretary-General of the United Nations, little has been done to alleviate this inequity. There are troublesome indications of the vaccine being used for economic and political gains. As I write this, Israel, a country with one of the highest rates of vaccinated citizens, has blocked the delivery of Russian manufactured vaccines to Gaza, and refused to vaccinate the millions of Palestinians living in the West Bank under Israeli occupation. Instead, Israel plans to share their surplus with countries in Africa and Latin America. This is just one example. The tragedy is that wide distribution of the vaccines throughout the world is what is required for vaccination to protect us all. The selfish shortsightedness of this unfair and unequal access to the available vaccines is unfathomable and potentially self-destructive.

Then there are the individuals who are making similarly self-ish and shortsighted decisions often based on limited or even false information. Many, all over the world, worry about taking the vaccine, uncertain about its safety given the rapidity of its development, the profit motives of pharmaceutical industries, and the history of scientific experimentation on certain populations throughout history. Conspiracy theories and false stories fill social media. If too many individuals make the decision to forego the vaccine, it will undermine the vaccination effort, and prevent the development of the widespread immunity required to control COVID-19.

Studies indicate that having and recovering from the virus seems to provide immunity for at least three months. The length of time that the vaccines provide protection is still uncertain, but seems to follow the pattern of influenza. That suggests that annual vaccines will need to be distributed prior to the COVID-19 season, much like we do for Flu season. However, exactly when that season is has yet to be determined. Then there are the variants: mutations that change the virus, and its communicability, its severity, the mortality rates, and even whether or not vaccines are protective, potentially making everything much worse. And we are only beginning to understand the plight of the long haulers who have persisting COVID symptoms for months.

Success depends on our willingness to mask, social distance, and limit large gatherings. The essential workers in the Chronicles were frustrated by the non-compliance they saw. Perhaps Dr. Anna said it best: "It's arrogant to not wear a mask." Personal rights and freedom versus the safety of society is a discussion we need to have in the US. Exercising the right to worship or gather in large groups has had devastating consequences. A September 2020, wedding reception with 55 guests in rural Maine lead to 177 COVID-19 cases, including seven hospitalizations and seven deaths (four who had been hospitalized). Our post-COVID world will likely continue its mask wearing, social distancing, and gathering limitations for awhile. We may be weary of the new rules, but the continued arrogance, ignorance, and non-compliance by a few will determine how quickly the US can move beyond COVID.

Countries like China, Korea, New Zealand and Australia have been more successful at controlling the spread of COVID. Understanding the components of their success will be the focus of future research, but on first blush, citizens in those countries worked together and followed guidelines; the welfare of all was prized above the freedom of a few. National leadership formed an organized response and used science to lay out guidelines.

The Black Lives Matter Movement brought to the foreground the gruesome realities of structural racism in the US. Jasmine said it best: "COVID makes everything harder. It magnifies the dysfunction" of racism in our society. COVID showed the inequity in health care, with more black and brown people dying. It highlighted the unfairness in employment, as low-wage essential workers, mostly people of color, risked their lives to deliver packages, clean health facilities, and produce food. This was often done as if they were dispensable, without adequate protection and without the enforcement of CDC safety and prevention guidelines. The injustice in housing and mortgage practices means unaffordable rents, necessitating crowded living in often unsafe neighborhoods. The list continues. These issues require public discussion and action.

Finding the resilience and strength to move forward...

Somehow, in spite of all the losses and challenges, the human spirit marches on. Jasmine said, "I am able to have a difficult moment and realize that I can rise above it. I cannot change it, it is what it is, and complaining and being depressed just makes it harder. I try to be positive... I start by really caring for and about people." Perhaps Jasmine is young and idealistic, but like many others in these Chronicles, she cares about and recognizes the humanity of her clients. Acknowledging our common vulnerabilities allows us to be kind and put our best selves forward. That includes knowing that we must make sacrifices for the health and safety of the community.

Dr. Jackie cares as well about her patients, coworkers, family, and community. When she grew disillusioned, she phoned her Grandma, whose wisdom and strength has been tempered by years of living in the rural south. Grandma listened and reminded her: "God is with you and it may take time, but it will work out." Both Jasmine and Dr. Jackie described faith as an anchor.

Dr. Miguel, Reed and others grounded themselves by being in and with nature. Living near the bay in Rhode Island where the Atlantic Ocean punches into the state creating several hundred miles of coastline, nature's power and tenacity is on display every day. I watch the ongoing drama of sky meeting water and the ebb and flow of the light and the tide. I've learned how the moon affects the tides and the life-cycle of the ancient-looking horseshoe crabs.

During the full moon every May, hundreds crawl out of the ocean to mate at the tideline on the sandy beach near my home. After several weeks, they disappear back into the water until the following May. They have followed the seasonal call for 300 million years, before dinosaurs inhabited the earth. They are a pertinent touch point here because scientists started caging them in the 1970s to harvest their unique and remarkable blue blood to check the safety of medicines. Most recently, it is used in the development of some COVID vaccines.

Find a reason to laugh…

Dr. Ben helped his COVID-testing newbies appreciate the very human response of having a swab jammed up your nose. Dr. Anna explained to the new resident how imperative humor was: "We can't be sad and depressed all the time." Jokes, stories, and anecdotes often poke fun at ourselves, family members, or pets—some silliness or embarrassment that we all have encountered. Nurse Susan was skilled at finding reasons to laugh and sharing her experiences in a way that made it easy to chuckle with her.

There is a physiologic benefit to laughter. At least a dozen facial muscles contract and the left and right sides of the brain communicate to make sense of what is said. Chemicals are released that lower stress hormones and boost our immune systems. Find an excuse to laugh at the insanity of it all.

Focus on gratitude and recognize the small delights…

Perhaps Fran, my special needs sister who recovered from COVID, may be the best example of staying focused on the present moment. Continuous gratitude is part of her personality. "Thanks for being my sister" and "Thanks for taking my call" are words I hear every time I talk with her. She did not need to take courses in mindfulness—it is just who she is.

The wisdom of the fool is an old story. Fran reminds me not to get too far ahead of myself, my worries or my problems—not to become too engaged in the gymnastics of my brain and scenarios that may never come to pass. Gratitude helps me appreciate what I think of as delights or de-lights. *De* is a Spanish preposition meaning "of" or "from." Gifts "of or from" the light. Gifts that brighten the dark times. When we pay attention, they are everywhere. We can appreciate the person who smiles, even behind the mask. The driver who allows us to butt in front of him in a busy lane of traffic. Sometimes they appear in unexpected places, like those red, yellow, and lavender wild flowers springing up amidst the trash scattered on the Palestinian hillside.

In-person visits are slowly starting up again. A three-day-old baby came in for a weight check just the other day. I spent a few extra seconds studying the infant who weighed in at just under six pounds—the miracle of his perfectly formed ears, ten fingers and ten toes, a strong suck on my gloved pinky finger. I cautiously fixed his diaper, scooped him up in his yellow-fleece blanket and handed him back to his smiling mother. "He's beautiful," I said, then slipped back into work mode and reviewed the follow up plan.

With careful attention to the moment, a day may offer a handful of delights. Sometimes I write them in my journal to capture and savor them. While this trudge through COVID, or what Dr. Irene called "Groundhog Day," may not become a two-step, the focused awareness on gratitude and the delights we encounter does lighten the burden of the mundane.

Treasure the family you have and create community...

In this time of isolation and pain, when friends and loved ones risk going to the hospital and disappearing but for the occasional glimpse on Zoom or FaceTime, our connections are more precious than ever. Whether the relationships are functional or dysfunctional, we are spending more time with people we live with. Maricela and Dr. Irene spoke of the support family gave them and worried how their exposure to COVID burdened their loved ones. Maricela and others made difficult choices about not visiting or including extended family members in celebrations in order to avoid and prevent COVID exposure.

Animals offer companionship and are four-legged family members. Dr Anna's cat received more attention than ever before. Drs. Miguel and his wife treasured the companionship of their dogs who were their excuse for getting outside.

For those without family in their households, it was imperative to find and create a community of support. Dr. Jackie reached out via social media, regularly phoned her Grandma, and connected with old friends and colleagues. Dr. Carla mailed packages ensuring that her friends felt loved.

Remember Self-Care...

When I search "self-care" on the internet, many nuggets appear from sages as varied as Buddha, Oprah, and Dolly Parton. Even Shakespeare who lived his entire life in the shadow of the Bubonic plague said in *King Henry V*: "Self-love, my liege, is not so vile a sin, as self-neglecting." Caregivers must care for themselves, otherwise they burn out. Dr. Carla gave special attention to this in her career. One of the silver linings of the pandemic for Dr. Jackie was more attention to her own self-care. Unfortunately, the workloads and the need to put food on the table and pay the rent, or employers with demands like Jasmine's, who ignored protocols, make self-care difficult if not impossible. For me, writing is part of my self-care—the opportunity to reflect and make sense of all that is happening around me and to me. Thanks for indulging me with your attention.

In closing, humans are resilient. The essential workers in these *Chronicles* put a foot forward and carried on, found opportunities for growth within the hardship of these turbulent times. Nature reminds us of the cycle of change and hope. The desert blooms after the winter rains and the sun rises every morning even if behind clouds.

It is only a matter of time until a new infectious agent or another novel virus appears and spreads in our global world. With climate change, the potential challenges are magnified and accelerated. Several years ago, an anthrax outbreak in Siberia was blamed on the defrosting of reindeer carcasses when the permafrost thawed. Anthrax spores had survived in reindeer herds thought to be killed by a plague nearly 100 years ago. Once melted, the microbes infected the reindeer and cattle grazing nearby that wandered into the area. No technology or walls can protect us from these kind of threats. Efforts exist to monitor where and when another virus might jump from its animal host to man, but these initiatives need to be expanded with more stable funding. Science and its findings need to be trusted and followed.

References

Quotations
John, J. "Shakespeare Quotes on the Coronavirus Pandemic." No Sweat Shakespeare. Last modified September 18, 2020. https://www.nosweatshakespeare.com/blog/shakespeare-quotes-on-the-coronavirus-pandemic/

Chapter 2
Mask recommendations & history
CDC. "Your Guide to Masks." COVID-19 Your Health. Last modified February 22, 2021. https://www.cdc.gov/coronavirus/2019-ncov/prevent-getting-sick/about-face-coverings.html
CDC. "Types of Masks." COVID-19 Your Health. Last modified February 23, 2021. https://www.cdc.gov/coronavirus/2019-ncov/prevent-getting-sick/types-of-masks.html
Wilson, Mark. "The untold origin story of the N95." Fast Company. March 24, 2020. https://www.fastcompany.com/90479846/the-untold-origin-story-of-the-n95-mask#:~:-text=By%20the%201970s%2C%20the%20Bureau,approved%20on%20May%2025%2C%201972

Jokes:
Beckerman, Jim. "Can jokes help cope with a pandemic? Coronavirus spawns dark humor." NorthJersey.com, June 17, 2020, https://www.northjersey.com/story/entertainment/columnists/jim-beckerman/2020/06/17/coping-with-coronavirus-pandemic-covid-19-spawns-dark-humor/5327568002/

PPE:

Hanage WP, Testa C, Chen JT, et al. COVID-19: US federal accountability for entry, spread, and inequities—lessons for the future. Eur J Epidemiol. 2020; 35:995-1006. https://doi.org/10.1007/s10654-020-00689-2

Chapter 3
Suicide:

Watkins, Ali Michael and Rothfeld, William K, et al. "Top E.R. Doctor Who Treated Virus Patients Dies by Suicide." New York Times. Updated April 29, 2020, https://www.nytimes.com/2020/04/27/nyregion/new-york-city-doctor-suicide-coronavirus.html

ICU:

Lapidus, N., Zhou, X., Carrat, F. et al. Biased and unbiased estimation of the average length of stay in intensive care units in the Covid-19 pandemic. Ann. Intensive Care. 2020;10:135. Published: 16 October 2020. https://doi.org/10.1186/s13613-020-00749-6

Chapter 4
COVID risk:

CDC. "Obesity, Race/Ethnicity, and COVID-19." Overweight & Obesity. Page last reviewed: January 8, 2021. https://www.cdc.gov/obesity/data/obesity-and-covid-19.html

Race/ethnicity:

CDC. "Risk for COVID-19 Infection, Hospitalization, and Death By Race/Ethnicity." COVID-19. Updated Feb. 18, 2021. https://www.cdc.gov/coronavirus/2019-ncov/covid-data/investigations-discovery/hospitalization-death-by-race-ethnicity.html

US COVID response:

Altman, Drew. "Understanding the US failure on coronavirus—an essay by Drew Altman." British Med Journal. 2020; 370:m3417. Published 14 September 2020. https://www.bmj.com/content/370/bmj.m3417

Diamond, Dan. "Inside America's 2-Decade Failure to Prepare for Coronavirus." POLITCO Magazine. Published April 1, 2020. https://www.politico.com/news/magazine/2020/04/11/america-two-decade-failure-prepare-coronavirus-179574

NH infections:

Fortier, Jackie. They Work In Several Nursing Homes To Eke Out A Living, And That May Spread The Virus. NPR. Published October 26, 2020

https://www.npr.org/sections/health-shots/2020/10/26/927841874/they-work-in-several-nursing-homes-to-eke-out-a-living-and-that-spreads-the-viru

Radiation experiments:

Markowitz G. The Treatment: The Story of Those Who Died in the Cincinnati Radiation Tests. Journal of American History. 2003; 90(1): 300–301. Published: June 01, 2003. https://doi.org/10.2307/3659917

NIH Scientist:

Bryant, Miranda. "Fauci praises African American scientist at 'forefront' of creating Covid vaccine." The Guardian. December 14, 2020. https://www.theguardian.com/world/2020/dec/14/kizzmekia-corbett-african-american-scientist-covid-vaccine

Chapter 10

Social determinants of health:

CDC. Social Determinants of Health: Know What Affects Health. Page last reviewed: January 26, 2021. https://www.cdc.gov/socialdeterminants/

Bandwidth:

Perrin, Andrew. Digital gap between rural and nonrural America persists. Pew Research Center. Published May 31, 2019. https://www.pewresearch.org/fact-tank/2019/05/31/digital-gap-between-rural-and-nonrural-america-persists/

Whitacre, Brian and Gallardo, Roberto. COVID-19 lockdowns expose the digital have-nots in rural areas - here's which policies can get them connected. The Conversation. Published September 2, 2020: https://theconversation.com/covid-19-lockdowns-expose-the-digital-have-nots-in-rural-areas-heres-which-policies-can-get-them-connected-144324

Primary care practice closure:

Ungar, Laura. Thousands of Doctors' Offices Buckle Under Financial Stress of COVID. KHN. Published November 30, 2020: https://khn.org/news/thousands-of-primary-care-practices-close-financial-stress-of-covid/

Burnout:

Templeton, K., C. Bernstein, J. Sukhera, L. M. Nora, C. Newman, H. Burstin, C. Guille, L. Lynn, M. L. Schwarze, S. Sen, and N. Busis. 2019. Gender-based differences in burnout: Issues faced by women physicians. NAM Perspectives. Discussion Paper, National Academy of Medicine, Washington, DC. https://doi.org/10.31478/201905a

Berg, Sara. Physician burnout: Which medical specialties feel the most stress. AMA News. Published January 21, 2020: https://www.ama-assn.org/practice-management/physician-health/physician-burnout-which-medical-specialties-feel-most-stress

Conclusion
New Zealand:
Boland, Billy. Billy Boland: How has New Zealand been so successful in managing covid-19? The BMJopinon. Published November 6, 2020: https://blogs.bmj.com/bmj/2020/11/06/billy-boland-how-have-new-zealand-been-so-successful-in-managing-covid-19/

Australia:
Blum, Jeremy. Fauci: Australia Has 'Done Actually Quite Well' Containing COVID-19, Unlike The U.S. HUFFPOST. Published October 28, 2020: https://www.huffpost.com/entry/fauci-australia-done-actually-quite-well-covid-19_n_5f99c-7fac5b61d63241edc23

Anthrax:
Timofeev V, Bahtejeva I, Mironova R, et al. Insights from Bacillus anthracis strains isolated from permafrost in the tundra zone of Russia. PLoS One. 2019;14(5):e0209140. Published: 19 May 2220. doi:10.1371/journal.pone.0209140

Maine wedding:
Mahale P, Rothfuss C, Bly S, et al. Multiple COVID-19 Outbreaks Linked to a Wedding Reception in Rural Maine — August 7–September 14, 2020. MMWR Morb Mortal Wkly Rep 2020;69:1686–1690. DOI: http://dx.doi.org/10.15585/mmwr.mm6945a5external icon

Israel block COVID vaccines:

Holmes, Oliver. Israel blocked Covid vaccines from entering Gaza, say Palestinians. The Guardian. Published February 16,202: https://www.theguardian.com/world/2021/feb/16/israel-blocked-covid-vaccines-from-entering-gaza-say-palestinians

ND. Israel freezes plan to send vaccines to foreign allies. ALJAZEERA. Published February 25, 2021: https://www.aljazeera.com/news/2021/2/25/israel-freezes-plan-to-send-vaccines-to-foreign-allies

Horseshoe Crabs:

Arnold, Carrie. Horseshoe crab blood is key to making a COVID-19 vaccine—but the ecosystem may suffer. National Geographic. Published July 2, 2020: https://www.nationalgeographic.com/animals/article/covid-vaccine-needs-horseshoe-crab-blood

Acknowledgments

Thanks to the essential workers who graced me with their stories. Participation in Nina Amir's Write Nonfiction in November Challenge helped me get on the right path for crafting this book. My appreciation to Reed Pike, Sandra Miller, Jesse Fenton and Angela Lehman for their content and editing guidance. Thanks to Valerie Duff-Strautmann for her fast-track copy-editing. Cheers to Jo Romer and Christel Brellochs for their eagle eyes and careful reading of the final draft.

Author Bio

Dr. Therese Zink is a family physician, teacher, researcher, and leader in family medicine. Her award-winning stories on doctoring have been published in literary and medical journals, and anthologies. Inspired by her work with patients, and alongside colleagues and students, Zink believes that listening to and holding the story are important components of healing. Understanding how our own stories intersect with others is crucial to personal and professional growth.

Other Works:

The Country Doctor Revisited: A 21st Century Reader (Kent State University, 2010). Stories, poems and essays about rural health care today written by rural health providers across the US.

Becoming a Doctor: Reflections by Minnesota Medical Students (University of Minnesota, 2011). A literary portrait of the many steps along the path to becoming a physician.

Confessions of a Sin Eater (2012). Zink's own stories that explore the privilege and burden of doctoring.

Mission Rwanda (2114)
Mission Chechnya (2017)
Dr. Ann McLannly Global Health Books
--Follow along with Dr. Ann who navigates landscapes and cultures during conflicts that garnered little media attention when they occurred. Like the Global Health volunteers enmeshed with forces beyond their control, your adrenaline will

pump as you become addicted to the intrigue, romance, and the challenge of practicing medicine on unfamiliar ground. Coming soon: Mission Cambodia

Website: http://www.theresezink.com/
Also on Linkedin and Facebook
Blog: https://www.theresezink.com/blog-tzinks-reflections/

www.ingramcontent.com/pod-product-compliance
Lightning Source LLC
Chambersburg PA
CBHW071702210326
41597CB00017B/2298